# Narrative Therapy with Spanish Speakers

*Narrative Therapy with Spanish Speakers* provides counselors, social workers, and other mental health professionals with a variety of culturally responsive bilingual activities developed for use with clients of all ages. Each short chapter covers topics such as fear, acceptance, and trust; the chapters also employ short fictions, sayings, and quotes, all in both Spanish and English, that professionals can share directly with clients. Additional materials on the book's website include audio resources for both counselors and clients, and the book is replete with icons and guides to help counselors quickly find relevant material.

**Roberto Swazo, Ph.D., PSL,** has been a professor and director of counseling at Roosevelt University, Florida Agricultural Mechanical University, and the University of Northern Iowa. He is a former Fulbright Scholar in Italy and licensed school counselor.

**Noelany Pelc, Ph.D.,** has been a director of online counseling programs and field clinical coordinator at Seton Hall University and is currently an assistant professor at Marian University. She is a licensed psychologist and educator.

# Narrative Therapy with Spanish Speakers

Creative Bilingual Strategies for Individual, Family, and Group Sessions

**Roberto Swazo and Noelany Pelc**

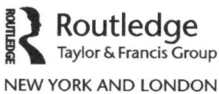
Routledge
Taylor & Francis Group

NEW YORK AND LONDON

**Cover image:** © Getty Images

First published 2023
by Routledge
605 Third Avenue, New York, NY 10158

and by Routledge
4 Park Square, Milton Park, Abingdon, Oxon, OX14 4RN

*Routledge is an imprint of the Taylor & Francis Group, an informa business*

© 2023 Roberto Swazo and Noelany Pelc

The right of Roberto Swazo and Noelany Pelc to be identified as authors of this work has been asserted in accordance with sections 77 and 78 of the Copyright, Designs and Patents Act 1988.

*Library of Congress Cataloging-in-Publication Data*
Names: Swazo, Roberto, author. | Pelc, Noelany, author.
Title: Narrative therapy with Spanish speakers : creative bilingual strategies
    for individual, family, and group sessions / Roberto Swazo and Noelany Pelc.
Description: New York, NY : Routledge, 2022. | Includes bibliographical references.
Identifiers: LCCN 2022007308 (print) | LCCN 2022007309 (ebook) |
    ISBN 9780367699505 (hardback) | ISBN 9780367699499 (paperback) |
    ISBN 9781003145943 (ebook)
Subjects: LCSH: Hispanic Americans—Mental health services. | Latin
    Americans—Mental health services—United States. | Narrative therapy. |
    Cross-cultural counseling. | Intercultural communication.
Classification: LCC RC451.5.H57 S93 2022 (print) | LCC RC451.5.H57 (ebook) |
    DDC 362.84/68073—dc23/eng/20220523
LC record available at https://lccn.loc.gov/2022007308
LC ebook record available at https://lccn.loc.gov/2022007309

ISBN: 978-0-367-69950-5 (hbk)
ISBN: 978-0-367-69949-9 (pbk)
ISBN: 978-1-003-14594-3 (ebk)

DOI: 10.4324/9781003145943

Access the companion website: narrativetherapybilingualstrategies.com

To the memory of my multilingual Sephardi family and ancestors.
Roberto (Gershon)

To all of the helpers who are tireless in seeking inspiration.
Noelany

# Contents

# About the Authors

Roberto Swazo, Ph.D.
University of Northern Iowa, Iowa

Dr. Swazo earned his bachelor's degree in general sciences and master's in school counseling from the University of Puerto Rico, and Ph.D. in counselor education from Oregon State University. Dr. Swazo has served as a school counselor in private and public schools, college counselor, and as a mental health consultant for private practice and non-profit organizations. He is a full professor at the school and mental health counseling program at the University of Northern Iowa (UNI), Cedar Falls, and has served as Program Director at Florida Agricultural and Mechanical University (FAMU) in Tallahassee, Florida; Roosevelt University (RU) in Chicago; and University of Northern Iowa, Cedar Falls. He currently holds a Professional Service License (PSL, K-12) in the state of Iowa.

In addition to teaching, Dr. Swazo is a frequent speaker at professional conferences and conducts workshops throughout the United States and abroad on multicultural issues and psycho-bilingual training (teaching basic Spanish interventions) for schools and mental health agencies. He has presented or has been invited as a keynote speaker in Mexico, Puerto Rico, Nicaragua, Guatemala, Costa Rica, Ecuador, Guatemala, Russia, Spain, Romania, Czech Republic, and Italy. He also teaches frequently as an invited professor at the Universidad del Valle in Guatemala in the school and mental health programs. He is a former Fulbright Scholar at the University of Palermo, Italy, where he lived for a period of time. Dr. Swazo is a dual citizen from the European Union (Spain) and the USA.

Books from Dr. Swazo:

Swazo, R. (2013). *The bilingual's counselor guide to Spanish: Basic vocabulary and interventions for the non-Spanish speaker*. Francis and Taylor: Routledge.
Swazo, R. (2021). *Fantasias e ilusiones desde el exilio* (Fantasies and illusions from the exile). (2nd ed., Spanish). Gershon Menashe Books.
Vernon, A., & Swazo, R. (2004). *Assessment interventions with children and adolescents: Developmental and cultural approaches*. American Counseling Association.

Noelany Pelc, Ph.D.
Marian University, Indiana

Dr. Noelany Pelc earned her bachelor's in psychology and master's in clinical psychology from Roosevelt University in Chicago, Illinois. During her training and post-graduation, she gained clinical experience working with womxn and children who were survivors of trauma and relational violence, particularly as those experiences intersected with marginalized and disenfranchised identities. She gained experience working with Latina community outreach and crisis intervention in the Chicagoland area of Illinois. Dr. Pelc earned her Ph.D. in counseling psychology from Texas Woman's University in Denton, Texas, focusing on feminist and multicultural issues. She gathered experience working with college counseling students, dual-diagnosis mental health concerns and cross-addiction within a residential setting, and training in psychological assessment for impaired professionals.

Dr. Pelc is a licensed psychologist in the state of New York and in Indiana, and previously served as the Clinical Coordinator for MA/EdS students in professional counseling and school counseling before serving as the Academic Director of the online School Counseling and Professional Counseling programs at Seton Hall University in New Jersey. Her current areas of research center on the experience of womxn in the academy; the socialization of polarized national attitudes; and applications of cultural humility in research, teaching, and mentorship. Her professional interests include relational-cultural theory, feminist theory, and pedagogy.

Recent publications from Dr. Pelc:

Pelc, N., Hasan, N. T., & Mollen, D. (2020). Feminist storytelling: Representing the stories of diverse women in psychology. *Women & Therapy, 43*, 1–17. https://doi.org/10.1080/02703149.2019.1684683

Pelc, N., & Mollen, D. (2020). Special issue conclusion: Representing the stories of diverse women in psychology. *Women & Therapy, 43.* https://doi.org/10.1080/02703149.2019.1684682

# Figures and Tables

## Figures

## Tables

# Acknowledgements

We would like to thank our dear editor Anna Moore for her dedication, professionalism, editorial wisdom, and most importantly for her patience and guidance during the last year.

To our spouses Chris and Dagmar for their patience and unconditional support. To Chris for his artistic and creative contributions.

Thanks to our graduate student Dana Marsden for her assistance and organization.

# Introduction

¡Hola! How many times have you thought about adding some spark to your traditional counseling interventions? And how many times have you thought about integrating basic principles of narrative therapy but ended up being stuck doing the same traditional interventions? You might have even contemplated the idea of integrating some multilingual activities but did not know where to start. It is likely that you also encountered some multilingual clients (English/Spanish) and you were experimenting with ways to pique their interest. Perhaps you have been waiting for some sort of exercise that could take into account the following ingredients: Spanish/English, culture, and counseling. This book contains all these elements and allows you to put your counseling skills into practice and the use of non-traditional therapies in an easy and culturally sensitive way. Perhaps your Spanish skills are not strong enough to establish a full and fluent conversation in Spanish; however, there is no need to do so with this book, as the microfictions, sayings, quotes, and morals, including the instructions for your clients, are provided in both languages. Now, if you are looking into expanding your Spanish repertoire and occasionally deviating from the instructions by adding your own Spanish *flavor* to the exercises, then we highly recommend you obtain a copy of *The Counselor's Guide to Spanish: Basic Vocabulary and Interventions for the Non-Spanish Speaker* (Swazo, 2013).

This book can be used in any mental health, community counseling, or private agency setting; school counseling or social work professional environment. If you want to challenge yourself and expand your knowledge base, the utilization of your high school or college level Spanish will serve as a great source of tools to enhance these interventions. Throughout this book you will find the Cultural Hints symbol pertaining to short cultural notes that provide information related to nuanced multicultural issues and how to prevent possible sources of confusion and discomfort. Also, along with the book you will find the instructions to access the Reader's Companion Website and the symbol indicating that these are narrated on the website. You can access the website using the following link: https://www.narrativetherapybilingual strategies.com/.

Although accents vary among Spanish speaking individuals, the essence of the Spanish language remains unaltered and communication among native speakers is very efficient. On the other hand, *broadcast*, or generic Spanish language, is used throughout this book, which is defined as a language free of cultural misinterpretations. Broadcast Spanish is typically used by Spanish speaking professionals in Latin America and is easily understood across native speakers (Weller, 1983).

DOI: 10.4324/9781003145943-1

## What Is Different About This Book From Others on the Market?

This book is designed with the professional counselors, psychologists, and social workers in mind—those who may understand some Spanish but are not fluent enough to conduct a full Spanish session by themselves without the assistance of extra resources or a translator. Additionally, this book can be used solely for English or Spanish speakers as it has all the necessary interventions and processing techniques in both languages. The book contains 22 original microfiction bilingual stories (micro cuentos) in conjunction with numerous sayings, quotes, and morals with key processing questions and exercises with non-traditional approaches to analyze and decode their content from a therapeutic stance. Stories have a unique way of connecting people's realities, fantasies, pains, miseries, and happiness. Instead of boring old tales that provoke drowsiness, these stories are meant to wake up and energize the reader. In essence, these microfictions, sayings, quotes, and morals are intended to provoke the client's need to think, self-reflect, and consequently alter thoughts, feelings, and behaviors that are not functioning well in their environments, for more effective ones.

In sum, it is an opportunity to conquer your linguistic fears and commence a new stage in your professional development. We invite you to an exciting linguistic and cultural voyage that will enhance your counseling skills and open the window to a new world. ¡Bienvenidos y adelante!

## How to Use This Book

In order to protect the authenticity of the original quotations, microfictions, morals, and sayings as they were written by the authors, the original gender designations have been kept as opposed to the utilization of more gender-neutral or gender-fluid terms. However, and as for any therapeutic tool, the counselor has the authority to alter the way these are told or expressed and can certainly be contextualized according to the needs or identity(ies) of the client(s). As an additional note, the Spanish language requires a gendered pronoun when referring to items, people, and so forth. Plural nouns default to masculine pronouns, unless the group is identifiably entirely female. These parts of speech are easily modifiable to best meet the needs and identity(ies) of the client(s).

This book has been purposely written from a non-theoretical posture in order to provide elasticity to practitioners to apply a myriad of possible techniques from their preferred theory or school of thought. Hence, counselors hold a moldable tool that can adapt to the needs of their client(s) based on their clinical judgement. Like any other therapeutic tool, the practitioner needs to know how to utilize it. There are some elements to be considered that could ensure a higher degree of success when utilizing this book.

### How to Access the Book Website and Recordings

You can access the Reader's Companion Website and contact the authors by utilizing the "Contact" feature. This communication is to verify purchase and access e-materials. You will have the opportunity to integrate the observations, listening skills, and cultural nuances, have access to electronic copies of tables presented, and be notified of new features or updates.

### Timing

The counselor must determine when the right time to use the microfiction, quotes, and sayings is. In other words, is your client ready to work or is the exercise building the therapeutic relationship between you? How much time do you have devoted to the activity? Do you have the right setting to implement the other extra exercises to process the content of the main activity? Do you need a co-therapist to work with you? Timing determines the effectiveness of an activity as long as the client is willing and able to be fully engaged and prepared for a more profound cognitive, emotional, and psychological quest for growth and development.

### Culture

The beauty of this book is that you can use one language or the other, exclusively, and it is not necessary to apply the bilingual concept. Or, you can use both languages in the same session as the material is already translated for you as a clinician. Keep in mind that people, regardless of their culture of origin, enjoy stories, sayings, quotes, and the teachings that can be derived from them. These are universal in nature! With that being said, always make sure that you can assess the level of comfort for your clients when implementing the exercises in case that you might run into cultural incompatibilities.

Similarly, while we offer some cultural hints and considerations, and draw on a range of morals, sayings, and quotes from numerous cultures, it is important to avoid generalizations or categorizations that promote assumptions about any group as a monolith. We recommend a focus on cultural humility and taking a stance of "not-knowing," wherein the client is the expert on their lives and there is an explicit acknowledgement of power differentials and cultural differences between clinicians and clients. The goal is to allow individuals to define themselves as they wish to do, and frame their own life stories, using the provided exercises as starting points.

### Gender

Since the microfictions are written using the original gender designations and pronouns, you might want to adapt gendered examples and language to the needs of your clients in order to increase the degree of relevance and avoid microaggressions. Likewise, quotes and sayings are being left intact without altering the original work but can easily be adapted to be more gender inclusive.

### Age

Developmentally appropriate interventions are key when working with all clients regardless of racial, ethnic, and cultural background. As a result, make sure that your client has the cognitive abilities and psychological and emotional maturity to comprehend the content of the exercises. Hence, you might want to do a quick assessment of content comprehension before engaging in a full activity.

### Modality

These exercises can be applied in traditional individual, group, and family counseling sessions including small groups or a teaching guidance lesson in a school environment. Additionally, some exercises can be used in couple's therapy by restructuring how the content is processed and by concentrating on presenting concerns of a singular participant or the relational unit. As a service provider, you have the flexibility of adapting contextually and recreating the scenarios to make it relevant to the clients and their needs.

## Socratic Questions and Critical Thinking

One of the key processing tools of this book is based on the use of Socratic questioning and critical thinking mechanisms. These must be used as a key therapeutic method in a non-invasive way replete with a sense of empathic curiosity. Questions are not meant to challenge the person but to explore the logic and rationale of the thinking process and generate movement. These questions will allow the client to examine preconceived ideas, concepts, personal preferences, principles, and beliefs to determine their level of validity, applicability, or value. Accordingly, the client can develop the ability to create a personal self-assessment system to continually identify harmful thinking processes in the absence of the counselor. In many ways, the counselor assists the client to become a more reflective examiner of closely held beliefs, ideas, and ways of engaging with the world.

## Narrative and Existential Counseling as a Foundation

In order to increase the level of effectiveness of this book and to minimize cultural biases while gravitating across cultures, this book relies on a range of theoretical platforms that are sensitive to the universal experiences of human beings as opposed to specific theoretical frameworks that are geared to members of a particular country or a specific sociocultural context. Existentialism and narrative therapy have an overarching umbrella ample enough to house the micro and macro human experiences from a cultural and linguistic perspective. All people rely on stories in order to promote their histories and cultures regardless of culture. Likewise, questioning one's origin and purpose in life is a transcendent trait that cuts across countries of origin and language. Hence, the following two sections provide a quick overview of the key principles from these two schools of thought and how they serve as the major lenses to work with your clients.

### Narrative Therapy

Have you noticed that most of our conversations are based on stories or short narratives? For instance, the following basic questions elicit stories that are summaries of subjective personal experiences: "How was your day? "Tell me about your summer trip." "Where did you grow up?" "Tell me about your childhood." "What do you remember the most about your parents?" Like these, there are common questions that elicit short or long narratives from us depending on the feelings associated with them. Then, by telling their stories, people assign meaning to these unique experiences and attempt to evaluate these issues that are being faced (White, 2007). As a result, these unique interpretations of the meanings associated with these stories allow individuals to create a sense of reality. Consequently, if the stories that people tell themselves have a negative connotation, these will have an impact on daily activities and interactions with others (Morgan, 2000). As a modality, narrative therapy is a social-emotional tool that allows individuals to modulate the internal experiences that generate pain and shape their worldview. Narrative therapy allows individuals to reframe and recontextualize experiences using a positive approach in order to create a more positive and productive story that leads to positive change.

In order to see the problems outside of themselves, clients are encouraged to externalize them to increase self-awareness and separate themselves from these problems (White, 2007). Narrative therapy is based on a non-judgemental process minimizing the individual to feel castigated by issues at hand. On the other hand, as individuals develop a sense of self-awareness, they learn to be accountable for their actions in different ways (Morgan, 2000). In general, narrative therapy is not overly concerned with diagnoses and sees the counselor as a healing guide during the therapeutic process. Narrative therapy is applicable across the vectors of age, class, gender, culture, race, and other dimensions of identity. By following the principles of narrative therapy, clients develop the tools to unpack and unravel their own personal stories with the intent of deconstructing negative elements and reconstructing or substituting these with positive ones. Key principles that are used throughout this book:

1. People's reality is socially constructed. Consequently, the client's interactions and dialogue with others impact the way their reality is experienced.
2. Reality is influenced by and communicated through language. This suggests that people who speak different languages may have radically different interpretations of the same experiences.
3. Having a narrative that can be understood helps us organize and maintain our reality. In other words, stories and narratives help us to make sense of our experiences.
4. There is no "objective reality" or absolute truth. What is true for us may not be the same for another person, or even for ourselves at another point in time.

(Standish, 2013)

In this book, you will see that clients are encouraged to re-tell certain stories in order to identify dominant narratives and assess their impact in their lives. In this era, clients are bombarded with hundreds of narratives via social media, TV, radio, and written media. Using narrative therapy strategies, clients are empowered to take control of their own stories and be their own narrators. Finally, modifying dominant narratives that are predominantly negative is achieved by using non-traditional counseling strategies such as art and music therapy principles, journaling, visualization, physical movement, meditation, and others.

*Existentialism Principles*

Existentialism is not a new therapeutic approach and by and large, it is based on philosophical principles rather than therapeutic principles. Existential therapy is the confluence between philosophy and therapy; moreover, it is a lifestyle and a way of thinking rather than just therapeutic principles. The philosophers who broke ground and created the foundation for the existential philosophy movement were Albert Camus (2006), Martin Heidegger (2000), Jean-Paul Sartre (2003), and Friedrich Nietzsche in Anderson (2006). Then, integrating the principles of existentialism and framing them into a therapeutic foundation, Irving Yalom (1980), Viktor Frankl (2006), and Rollo May (1981) created a set of operationalized principles that combated the vagueness and, at times, seemingly unreachable principles of the philosophical existential elements into a more practical approach. In general, the existential approach to therapy emphasizes the following six propositions (Frankl, 2006):

1. All persons have the capacity for self-awareness.
2. As free beings, everyone must accept the responsibility that comes with freedom.
3. Each person has a unique identity that can only be known through relationships with others.
4. Each person must continually recreate themselves. The meaning of life and of existence is never stagnant; instead, it evolves frequently.
5. Anxiety is part of the human condition.
6. Death is a basic human condition that gives significance to life.

One of the advantages of the existential therapy approach is that it allows clients to approach several dimensions such as the physical, social, psychological, and spiritual. Thus, instead of using a more mechanistic approach to changing the cognitive processes with the eventual goal of altering the behavior, the combination of narrative and existential schools encompasses a broader approach to helping individuals from all cultures.

## Basic Definitions

The following definitions provide a platform for the reader and practitioner to understand the power of these literary tools and their adaptation to a psychological environment such as counseling or therapy.

### Microfictions

*Microfiction* is a loose term typically ascribed to very short stories. Sometimes they are referred to as nanofictions, ministories, or flash fiction. In essence there is no authoritative definition for these types of condensed stories, but the overall consensus is that unlike in a long story or a novel, characters are not fully described, events are superficially explored, and elaboration of a plot is minimal. The essence or message of the story takes precedence over any other elements, allowing the reader to fill the gaps and redesign the characters, context, and plot with the final intent of drawing unique meaning based on one's emotional, psychological, spiritual, and cultural needs.

### Morals

*Morals* are a type of narrative that involves a lesson that challenges the listeners or readers to analyze a situation, event/experience, or interaction in order to derive personal meaning out of it. Ultimately, the intent of the moral is to invite the readers to recontextualize the main challenge of the story to their lives and make subjective determinations of what is right or correct, for them. Morals invite readers to evaluate their personal moral compasses and explicate why they act the ways that they act under certain circumstances. Then, morals are centered on a series of questions such as: (a) is this the right thing to do?, (b) if I behave in a certain manner versus another way, what are the consequences of my actions?, and (c) what is motivating me to think, feel, and act this way?

## *Sayings*

Sayings are concise or compact expressions that are packed with penetrating wisdom, and many times are accompanied with direct or indirect advice. On occasion, sayings are anchored in a rich cultural context that mimics the passing of historical events that have been intrinsically absorbed throughout the years. These economic expressions underscore formulations of basic truths or propositions that serve as an apparatus for beliefs that will guide critical thinking, logic, and reasoning. Frequently, sayings communicate a specific objective, proposition, or a general idea. Sayings transcend the specificity of a culture as these have been the preferred teaching vehicles of oral cultures across the globe.

## *Quotes*

In its basic nature, a *quote* is a piece of transcription of what someone said or wrote. In essence, the central aspect of a quote is that someone is repeating verbatim a message said or written by an individual, which should remain unaltered and credit must be given to its original author. Quotes can be conceptualized as tidbits of wisdom as proclaimed by someone who has had unique life experiences, education, revelations, and insights. Then, the reader or listener becomes a recipient of inspiration in order to rectify certain behaviors, reset personal goals, develop empathy, or simply be inspired.

## References

Anderson, R. L. (2006). Nietzsche on strength and achieving individuality. *International Studies in Philosophy*, *38*(3), 89–115.

Camus, A. (2006). *The fall*. Penguin.

Frankl, V. (2006). *Man's search for meaning*. Beacon Press.

Heidegger, M. (2000). *Introduction to metaphysics*. Yale University Press.

May, R. (1981). *Man's search for himself*. W. W. Norton Company.

Morgan, A. (2000). *What is narrative therapy: An easy-to-read introduction*. Dulwich Centre Publications.

Sartre, J. P. (2003). *Being and nothingness*. Routledge.

Standish, K. (2013, November 8). *Lecture 8: Introduction to narrative therapy*. Slideshare. www.slideshare.net/kevins299/lecture-8-narrative-therapy

Swazo, R. (2013). *The bilingual counselor's guide to Spanish: Basic vocabulary and interventions for the non-Spanish speakers*. Francis and Taylor: Routledge.

Weller, G. (1983). The role of language as a cohesive force in the Hispanic speech community of Washington. D.C. In L. Elias-Olivares (Ed.), *Spanish in the U.S. setting: Beyond the Southwest*. National Clearinghouse for Bilingual Education. Rosslyn, VA: Inter American Research Associates.

White, M. (2007). *MAPS of narrative practice*. W.W. Norton & Company.

Yalom, I. Y. (1980). *Existential psychotherapy*. Basic Books.

# Part I

# Relationships

Self and Others

# 1  Relationships

Relationships are one of the pillars of humanity that starts from the interaction between two individuals and grows into families, communities, societies, nations, and a higher being(s) for those who pursue spirituality. As a result, understanding the complex dynamics of relationships is key in order to succeed in life, intimacy, family, careers, and society at large. Those who master the art of forming healthy relationships pave the way for more meaningful relationships with fewer moments of conflict and periods of disconnection. On the contrary, those who go through life leaving a destructive path of toxic interactions become emotionally and psychologically ill and dysfunctional. A great number of clients who seek out clinical mental health services come to us with a history of broken relationships that have damaged many people and have been the cause of self-destructive patterns of behavior. Evaluation of current and past relationships is always a good start to a healthy way of correcting broken patterns of interaction that leads to self-respect.

Also see: forgiveness, humility and self-compassion, change and death and grief

 ## Microfiction

### Disconnected

Under the tenuous lamp's light, surrounded by the dark and penetrating silence of the living room, I crashed on the sofa. I started perusing dozens of texts and emails from my email inbox. These are old and recent ones, just as if I were reading a collection of short letters by many people who intersected with my life at some point in time. Various themes emerged from the texts and emails: recrimination, discontent, demands, putdowns, ignoring, harassing, detestation, hatred, contempt, making fun of, rejection, apathy, indifference, and envy. My parents passed away but kept their distance from me even during their last days at the senior center. My siblings have not communicated with me for over a decade. Since the divorce, all my children have cut off communication as my ex-spouse did. Other family members have avoided me like the plague since the last altercation. After the last shouting match with my neighbors due to their children's interest in my backyard, I have been ignored as if I didn't exist. At work, well, it's work. They are just coworkers who are forced to talk to me because of the projects to be completed. Friends? I am not sure if the friends from my childhood count. I have no clue where they ended up. After all, they disliked my arrogance and disdain, so they said back then. Intimacy, relationships? An emptiness invades my soul.

*(Español)*

DOI: 10.4324/9781003145943-3

## Microficción

### Desconectado

*Bajo la tenue luz de la lámpara, rodeado por el silencio oscuro y penetrante de la sala de estar, me caí en el sofá. Comencé a leer decenas de mensajes de texto y correos electrónicos desde mi bandeja de entrada. Estos son viejos y recientes, como si estuviera leyendo una colección de cartas cortas de muchas personas que se cruzaron con mi vida en algún momento determinado. Varios temas surgieron de los textos y correos electrónicos: recriminación, descontento, demandas, humillaciones, ignorar, hostigamiento, detestar, odio, desprecio, burla, rechazo, apatía, indiferencia y envidia. Mis padres fallecieron pero mantuvieron su distancia de mí incluso durante sus últimos días en el centro para personas mayores. Mis hermanos no se han comunicado conmigo durante más de una década. Desde el divorcio, todos mis hijos cortaron la comunicación al igual que mi ex cónyuge. Otros miembros de la familia me evitan como la plaga desde el último altercado que tuvimos. Después del último altercado e intercambio de gritos con mis vecinos debido al interés de sus hijos en el patio trasero de mi casa, me ignoran como si no existiera. En el trabajo, bueno, es trabajo. Son solo compañeros de trabajo que se ven obligados a hablar conmigo debido a los proyectos que se completarán. ¿Amigos? No estoy seguro si los amigos de mi infancia cuentan. No tengo idea de dónde terminaron. Después de todo, no les gustaba mi arrogancia y mi desdén, por lo que dijeron en aquel entonces. ¿Intimidad, relaciones? Un vacío invade mi alma.*

Author: Roberto Swazo.

### Cultural Hints

Disconnection and loneliness is a global issue. Remember to evaluate if the disconnection is a result of a natural disaster, war, or forced emigration as opposed to the resulting consequences of the client's negative behaviors. Northern Europeans stress independence and geographical distance, in contrast with South European/Mediterranean, Middle Eastern, and African cultures that underscore the importance of group intimacy. Hence, the subjective experience of the individual must be assessed to differentiate cultural versus personal traits.

### Processing questions for the clients (Preguntas de proceso para los/as clientes)

1. What do you think is going on with the main character? Explain. (*¿Qué crees que está pasando con el personaje principal? Explica.*)
2. Can you relate to them? If not, what kind of feelings is this person experiencing? Make a list of these feelings. (*¿Puedes relacionarte con él? Si no, ¿por qué tipo de sentimientos está pasando esta persona? Haz una lista de estos sentimientos.*)
3. Look at the picture that follows. In what way does this picture represent the mental state and life of this person? How many times have you felt like you have been clashing with everybody around you? Whose fault is it? Elaborate. (*Mira la foto de abajo. ¿De qué manera esta imagen representa el estado mental y la vida de esta persona? ¿Cuántas veces te has sentido como si estuvieras chocando con todos a tu alrededor? ¿De quién es la culpa? Elaborar.*)

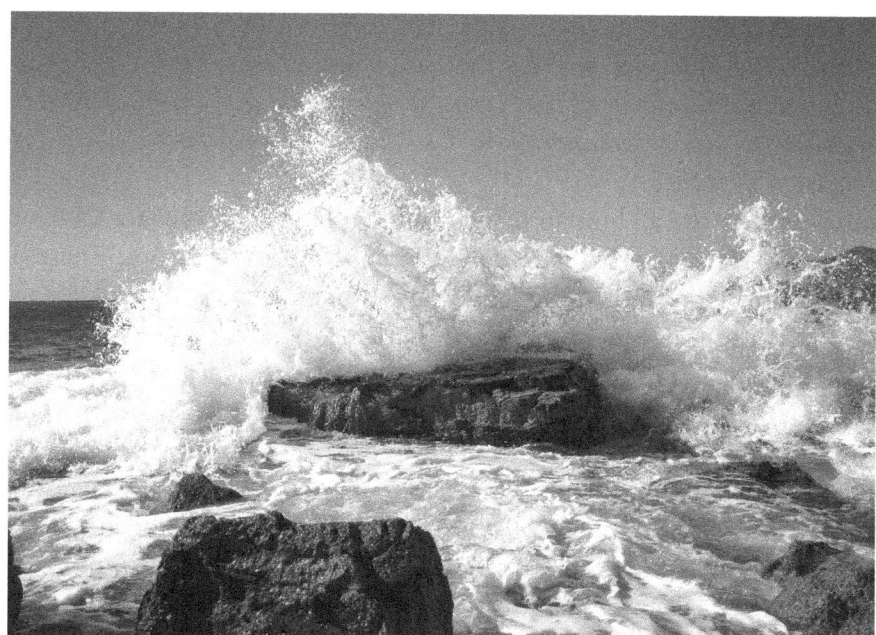

*Figure 1.1* Waves Crashing on Sea Rocks

## Sayings (*dichos*)

### *Saying #1*

"Relationships are like a vineyard, they are cultivated, cared for and maintained, then later enjoyed like good wine."

*"Las relaciones son como el viñedo, se cultivan, cuidan y mantienen para luego disfrutarlas como el buen vino."*

Author: Unknown. Popular Spaniard saying (V. Romero, personal communication, December 14, 2020).

**Processing questions for the clients (Preguntas de proceso para los/as clientes)**

1. Have you ever planted anything that bore fruit? Be it vegetables or fruits, what are the main characteristics of the entire process since you planted the first seed on the ground? Describe it. How does the issue of time and dedication in order to reap the benefits compare to your relationships? (*¿Alguna vez has plantado algo que dio frutos? Ya sean vegetales o frutas, ¿cuáles son las principales características de todo el proceso desde que plantaste la primera semilla en el suelo? Describelo. ¿Cómo se compara la cuestión del tiempo y la dedicación para madurar los beneficios con tus relaciones?*)

2. The following is a list of strategies to "cultivate" your relationship like a plant in such a way that you can later enjoy its wonderful "fruits." (*La siguiente es una lista de estrategias para "cultivar" tu relación como una planta de tal manera que luego puedas disfrutar de sus maravillosas "frutos".*)

a. Among many other things, make sure that a determined number of relationships is your priority. List the relationships that you want as a priority in order to enjoy them in the future. (*Entre muchas otras cosas, asegúrate de que un número determinado de relaciones sea tu prioridad. Enumera las relaciones que deseas como prioridad para disfrutarlas en el futuro.*)

b. Remember that we are all human beings and that in spite of the fact that you are making these relationships a priority, it is possible that others might not. Therefore, there are some disappointments in the process. Always remember how difficult it is to keep a plant healthy! (*Recuerda que todos somos seres humanos y que a pesar de que estás haciendo de estas relaciones una prioridad, es posible que otros no. Por lo tanto, hay algunas decepciones en el proceso. ¡Recuerda siempre lo difícil que es mantener una planta saludable!*)

c. In spite of being disillusioned at times, avoid insulting and recriminating those that you care about. Remember that when your plant looks weak, dry, and tiny you do not stop watering or nurturing it! On the contrary, that is the time to invest in its care. (*A pesar de a veces estar desilusionado, evita insultar y recriminar a aquellos que te importan. ¡Recuerda que cuando tu planta se ve débil, seca y pequeña, no dejes de regarla o cuidarla! Por el contrario, ese es el momento en que la cuidas más.*)

d. Resist blaming others for failures in the relationship. Look deep and see what you can change to adapt and make this relationship a successful one. (*Resiste culpar a otros por fallas en la relación. Mira profundamente y ve qué puedes cambiar para adaptarte y hacer que esta relación sea exitosa.*)

e. Resist trying to change others; each person is in charge of their lives. Your job is to work on you and keep sustaining others. Just like the time that is invested in a plant. (*Resiste el cambiar a los demás, cada persona es responsable de su vida. Tu tarea es trabajar contigo mismo y sostener a los demás. Así, como con el tiempo invertido en una planta.*)

f. Concentrate and focus on all the positives and good attributes from those around you. A strengths-based approach is healthy and uplifting. (*Concéntrate y enfócate en todos los aspectos positivos y buenos atributos de quienes te rodean, un enfoque basado en las fortalezas es saludable y estimulante.*)

3. Let's engage in a guided imagery exercise. Close your eyes, breath in and out for 2 minutes. Let your muscles relax and just concentrate on your breathing, forget about everything around you or close to you. Forget about other responsibilities or duties, just be in the present and allow your body to release the stress it is holding. Now, imagine a scenario in which there is tension with the person that you are trying to establish or repair the relationship with. Visualize the place, location, environment, and any other detail that represents the context of interaction. Picture as if this person's voice volume is being amplified.

These are the steps you have to take; simply construct these in your mind and be ready to enact them understanding the product will be positive: (*Realicemos un ejercicio de imágenes guiadas. Cierra los ojos, inhala y exhala por dos minutos. Deja que tus músculos se relajen y concéntrate en tu respiración, olvídate de todo lo que te rodea o está cerca de ti. Olvídate de otras responsabilidades o deberes, simplemente estás en el presente y libera tu cuerpo del estrés que lo está presionando. Ahora, imagina un escenario en el que hay tensión con la persona con la que estás tratando de establecer o reparar la relación. Visualiza el lugar, la ubicación, el entorno y cualquier otro detalle que represente el contexto de interacción. Imagínate a esta persona elevando el volumen de la voz.*

*Estos son los pasos que debes seguir, simplemente constrúyelos en tu mente y prepárate para implementarlos, entendiendo que el producto será positivo:)*

a. Pay close attention to the person's non-verbals, mannerisms, voice, eye contact, etc. (*Presta mucha atención a los no verbales, gestos, voz, contacto visual, etc. de la persona.*)

b. Attempt to recognize or pinpoint the patterns of communication of this person in front of you. (*Intenta reconocer o identificar los patrones de comunicación de esta persona que está frente a ti.*)

c. Take a glance at your past reactions, how you have reacted, what went well and what did not. Remember the way you talked, unproductive words and mannerisms that served as unwanted triggers. And, recall all the positive elements of interaction that can be replicated again. (*Echa un vistazo a tus reacciones pasadas, cómo has reaccionado, qué salió bien y qué no. Recuerda la forma en que hablaste, palabras improductivas y gestos que sirvieron como desencadenantes no deseados. Y recuerda todos los elementos positivos de interacción que pueden ser replicados nuevamente.*)

d. Exercise empathy and force yourself to feel and think the way the other person does. (*Ejercita la empatía y esfuérzate por sentir y pensar como lo hace la otra persona.*)

e. After all these, express how you feel and be sensitive to the needs of the other person. (*Después de todo esto, expresa cómo te sientes y sé sensible a las necesidades de la otra persona.*)

f. Evaluate the outcome, fix what's needed, and repeat the process again. (*Evalúa el resultado, arregla lo que se necesita y repite el proceso nuevamente.*)

## Saying #2

"Who did not look for friends in joy that in misfortune does not ask for them."
*"Quien no buscó amigos en la alegría que en la desgracia no los pida."*

Author: Unknown. Popular Latin American saying (S. Mendez, personal communication, February 1, 2017).

## Processing questions for the clients (Preguntas de proceso para los/as clientes)

1. What is your interpretation of this quote? Can you think of a time in your life that reflects the meaning of this quote? Explain. (*¿Cuál es tu interpretación de esta cita? ¿Puedes pensar en un momento de tu vida que refleje el significado de esta cita? Explique.*)

2. How many friends have you had in your life? At what stages of your life did these people share their journey with you? Name some of those that you are still in contact with and what you can do to replicate the same success? (*¿Cuántos amigos has tenido*

*en tu vida? ¿En qué etapas de tu vida estas personas compartieron su viaje contigo? Menciona algunos de los que todavía están en contacto y, ¿qué puedes hacer para replicar el mismo éxito?)*

3.  Describe the picture that follows. What do you think they are going through? Have you ever experienced these emotions? Explain. (*Describe la imagen de abajo. ¿Por qué crees que ellos están pasando? ¿Alguna vez has experimentado estas emociones? Explica.*)

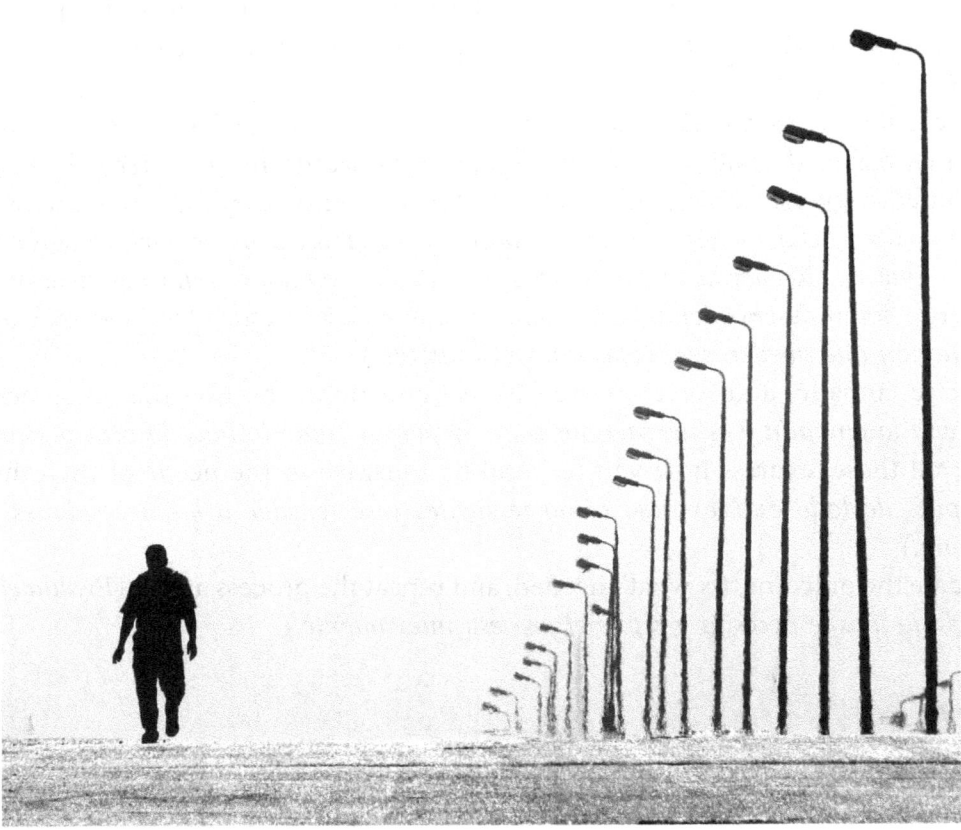

*Figure 1.2* Man Walking Alone

## Quotes

### *Quote #1*

"Honest communication is built on truth and integrity and respect for one another."
   "*La comunicación honesta está construida en la verdad e integridad y en el respeto del uno por el otro.*"

Author: Benjamin E. Mays, American Baptist minister and civil rights leader who is credited with elements of the intellectual foundations of the Civil Rights Movement (Ivy, 1961).

**Processing questions for the clients (Preguntas de proceso para los/as clientes)**

1. Can you provide examples in which you have violated the truth and integrity of a relationship? What were the consequences? What have you learned? (*¿Puedes dar ejemplos en los que hayan quebrantado la verdad y la integridad de una relación? ¿Cuáles fueron las consecuencias? ¿Qué has aprendido?*)

2. Describe the picture that follows. What is your interpretation? (*Describe la imagen de abajo. ¿Cuál es tu interpretación?*)

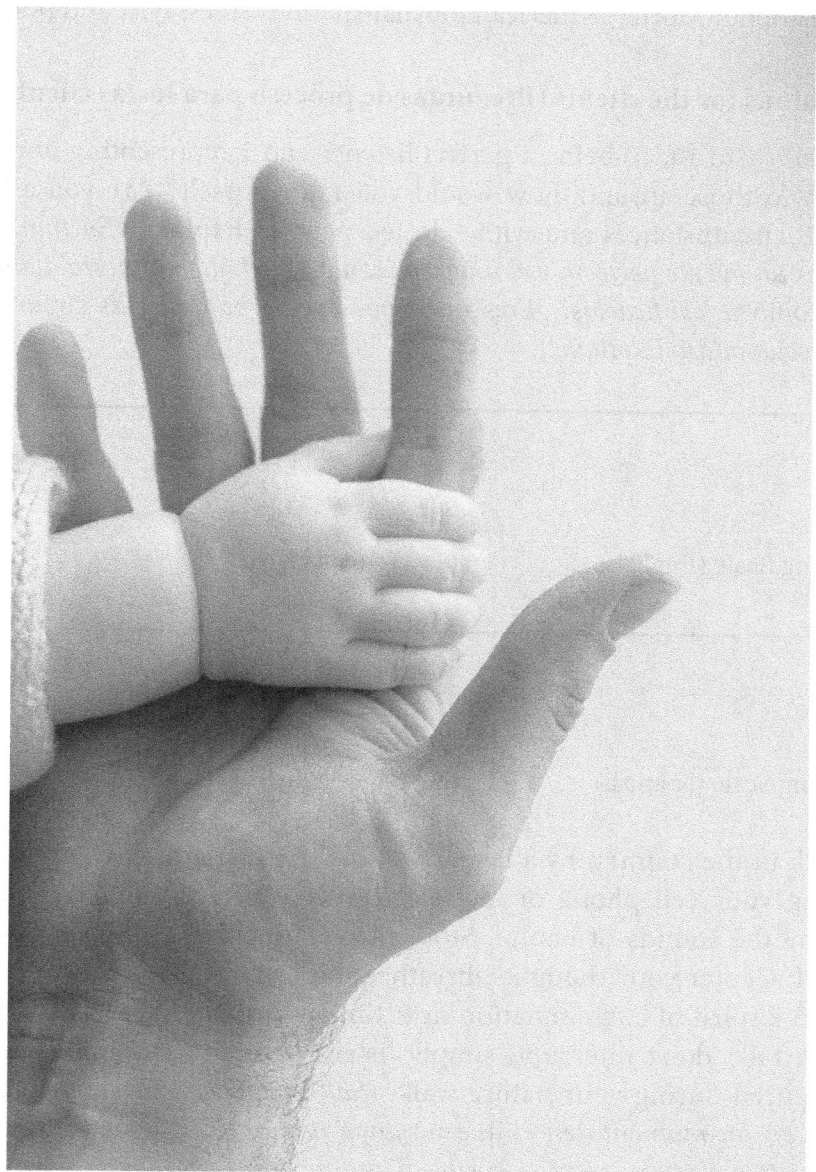

*Figure 1.3* Holding Hands

3. Make a list of songs that reinforce the idea of forgiving. Ask the same of the person that you are building a relationship with and compare the lists of songs. Process the lists with each other. (*Haz una lista de las canciones que refuerzan la idea de perdonar. Haz la misma*

*pregunta a la persona con la que estás construyendo una relación y compara la lista de canciones. Procesen la lista entre ustedes.)*

### Quote #2

"There is only one rule to be a good communicator; learn to listen."
   *"Solo hay una regla para ser un buen comunicador; aprender a escuchar."*

Author: Christopher Morley, American journalist, novelist, essayist and poet (2021).

### Processing questions for the clients (Preguntas de proceso para los/as clientes)

1. On a scale from 1 to 10, 10 being a perfect listener and 1 representing one who does not pay attention to those around, how would you rate yourself? Are you a better listener under certain circumstances and with selected people? Explain. (*En una escala del uno al diez, diez es un oyente perfecto y el uno representa aquel que no presta atención a quienes lo rodean, ¿cómo te calificarías? ¿Eres un mejor oyente bajo ciertas circunstancias y con personas seleccionadas? Explique.*)

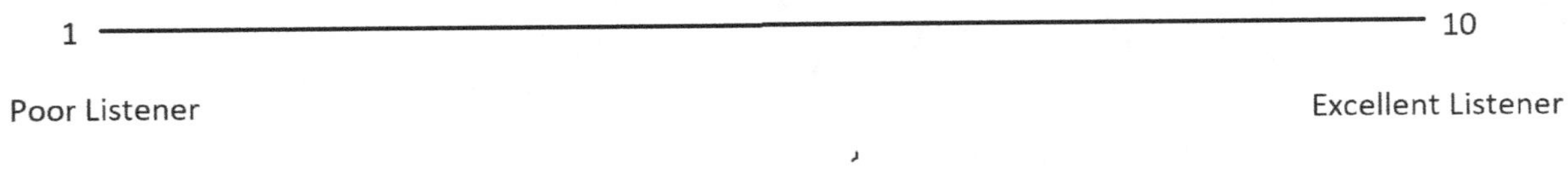

1 ——————————————————————————————— 10

Poor Listener                                        Excellent Listener

*Figure 1.4* Listening Scale (English)

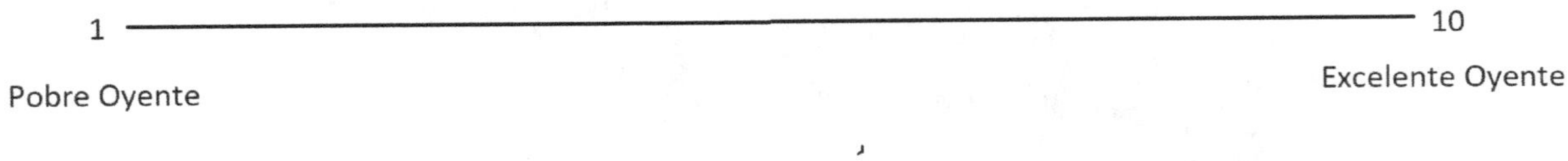

1 ——————————————————————————————— 10

Pobre Oyente                                         Excelente Oyente

*Figure 1.5* Listening Scale (Spanish)

2. Go for a walk in the country, by a lake, river, or a park at a time where there is no one. Do not bring your cell phone or any electronic device, if able. Walk leisurely, look around, enjoy the sounds of nature. Stop, sit on the grass, close your eyes, reconnect with yourself. Center your thoughts, breathe, and learn to be quiet for the time being. Bring the same spirit of contemplation next time when you have a conversation; let the other person talk, don't interrupt, simply listen. Maintain the inner peace of silence that you acquired during your nature walk. (*Sal a caminar por el campo, el lago, el río o un parque en un momento en el que no haya nadie. No traigas tu teléfono celular ni ningún dispositivo electrónico, si es posible. Camina tranquilamente, mira a tu alrededor, disfruta de los sonidos de la naturaleza. Detente, siéntate en la hierba, cierra los ojos, vuelve a conectarte contigo mismo. Centra tus pensamientos, respira y aprende a estar callado por el momento. Trae contigo el mismo espíritu de contemplación la próxima vez que tengas una conversación, deja que la otra persona hable, no interrumpas, simplemente escucha. Mantén la paz interior de silencio que adquiriste durante tu caminata por la naturaleza.*)

3. Apply the basic principle of empathy next time you a verbal disagreement brewing with someone, especially with those whom you are attempting to build a relationship. Put yourself in the shoes of the other person and imagine what they are thinking about you. Experience their sensations and emotions. Then, calibrate your communication tone. It is likely that you will understand then why this person is irritated by your prevalent attitudes. What does the picture that follows say about empathy? (*Aplica el principio básico de empatía la próxima vez que estés a punto de tener una discusión con alguien, especialmente con aquellos con los que estás tratando de construir una relación. Ponte en el lugar de la otra persona e imagina lo que él/ella está pensando en ti. Experimenta sus sensaciones y emociones. Luego, calibra tu tono de comunicación. Es probable que entiendas por qué esta persona está irritada por tus actitudes prevalentes. ¿Qué dice la siguiente imagen sobre la empatía?*)

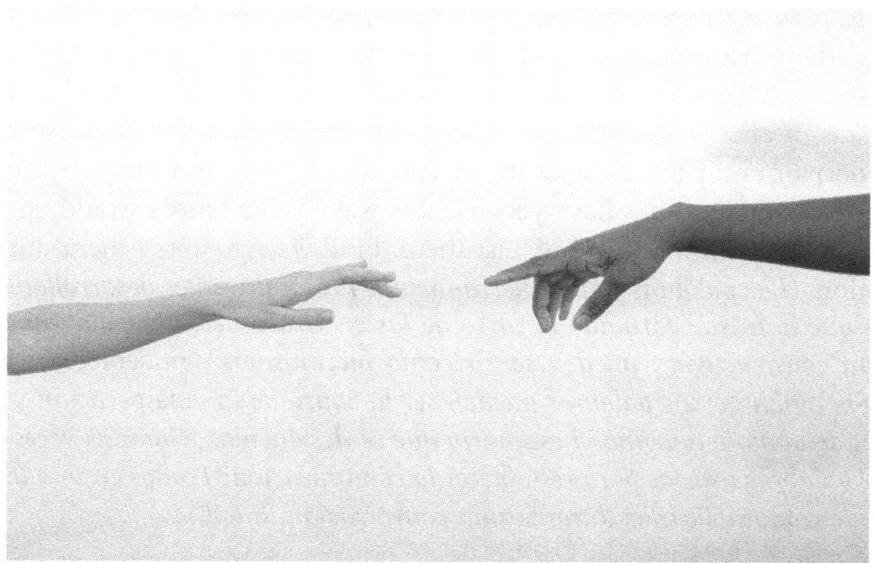

*Figure 1.6* Hands Reaching Out to Touch

### Quote #3

"You never know when a moment and a few sincere words can have an impact on a life."
   "*Nunca sabes cuando un momento y unas pocas palabras sinceras pueden tener un impacto en una vida.*"

Author: Zig Ziglar, American author, salesman, and motivational speaker (2014).

### Processing questions for the clients (Preguntas de proceso para los/as clientes)

1. What are sincere words to you? Have you been on the receiving end of these in your life? Cite examples. (*¿Qué son palabras sinceras para ti? ¿Has estado en el extremo receptor de estos en tu vida? Citar ejemplos.*)
2. Take a big cardboard piece, drawing, or sketching paper from a roll. Use washable tempera paint and use it to manifest your frustration about your current relationships. What do

the colors represent? Did you use each one on purpose? Are you mixing them up or keeping specific separation of colors? Let them dry and use words that represent them. On a separate, big cardboard piece, large drawing paper, or sketching paper from a roll, repeat the exercise now but with the intent to repair these relationships. Mix colors in such a way that the outcome represents your hopeful view of these relationships. Let them dry and use nurturing and positive words to represent them. (*Toma un pedazo grande de cartón, papel de dibujo grande o papel de boceto de un rollo. Usa pintura de témpera lavable y úsala para manifestar tu frustración sobre tus relaciones actuales. ¿Qué representan los colores? ¿Usaste cada uno a propósito? ¿Los estás mezclando o manteniendo una separación específica de colores? Déjalos secar y usa palabras que los representen. En una pieza de cartón grande separada, papel de dibujo grande o papel de boceto de un rollo, repite el ejercicio ahora pero con la intención de reparar estas relaciones. Mezcla colores de tal manera que el resultado represente tu visión esperanzadora de estas relaciones. Déjalos secar y usa palabras enriquecedoras y positivas para representarlos.*)*

3.  Words are the most influential tools developed by human beings that have transformed the course of civilizations. Words can be used in a constructive way and can serve as mechanisms of encouragement, revelation, and idealization. However, words can be the cause of despair and pain. Look at the picture that follows and imagine the scenario that unfolded. How many times have you felt this way? What words would you use in order to reestablish the communication? List them. Find ways to apply them during a difficult conversation. (*Las palabras son las herramientas más influyentes desarrolladas por los seres humanos que han transformado el curso de las civilizaciones. Las palabras pueden usarse de manera constructiva y pueden servir como mecanismos de aliento, revelación e idealización. Sin embargo, las palabras pueden ser la causa de la desesperación y el dolor. Mira la imagen de abajo e imagina el escenario que se desvincula. ¿Cuántas veces te has sentido así? ¿Qué palabras usarías para restablecer la comunicación? Ponlos en una lista. Encuentra maneras de cómo aplicarlos durante una conversación difícil.*)

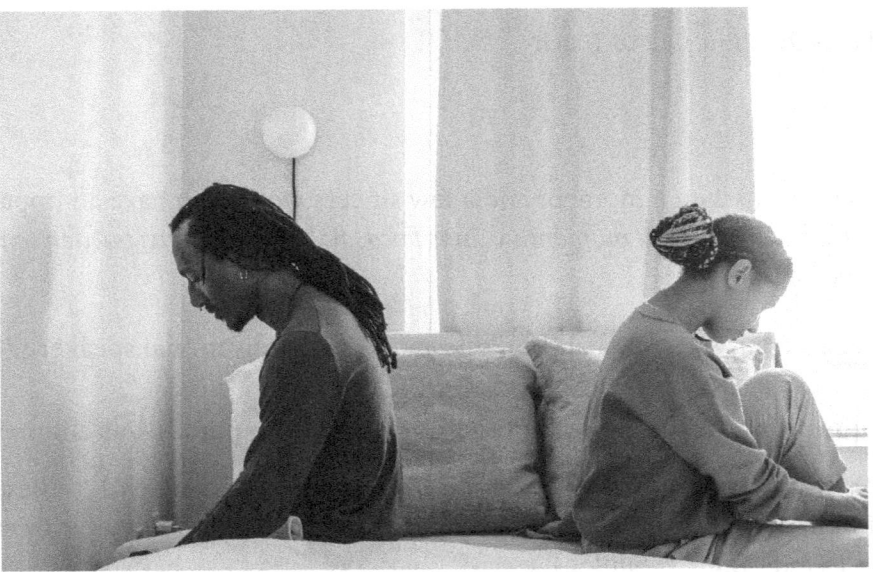

*Figure 1.7* Couple Sitting on a Bed Facing Away From Each Other

# References

Ivy, J. W. (1961, January). *A Record of the darker races*. The Crisis. https://books.google.com/books?id=6FsEAAAAMBAJ&lpg=PA27&ots=oFBW0FC89t&dq=when%20did%20benjamin%20mays%20say%20honest%20communication&pg=PA1#v=onepage&q=when%20did%20benjamin%20mays%20say%20honest%20communication&f=false

Morley, C. (2021, April 17). www.quotenova.net/authors/christopher-morley/xd7de5

Ziglar, Z. (2014, December 5). You never know when a moment and a few sincere words can have an impact on a life. [Image attached] [Status update]. *Facebook*. www.facebook.com/ZigZiglar/posts/10152899497167863:0

# 2   Trust

Trust is a central component of how individuals see themselves, engage with others, and relate to broader institutions around them. Trust exists in various realms, including as an internal experience, where self-efficacy, trust in one's decision-making, and confidence reside. It is also often discussed in relationships and the capacity to trust others. Trusting others requires beliefs and ideas about how others will act and behave in relationships. Similarly, trust is extended to the therapeutic relationship, when seeking medical care, when working with colleagues, and when engaging with neighbors, friends, family, and larger systems (e.g., government, organizations).

Trust is rarely absolute but rather is moderated and restricted by particular situations and carries emotional ties and associations. Individuals who explore these dimensions of trust can cultivate a greater sense of self-efficacy, develop acceptance of their own choices, foster meaningful relationships with others in ways that are safe, and critically examine how they relate to broader systems in their day-to-day lives.

Also see: relationships, identity and liberation, change, courage and peace

## Cultural Hints

Trust in institutions, political groups, healthcare systems, community policing, and other major systems can vary drastically according to the client's identities and intersectionalities. Distrust and skepticism may have emerged as an adaptive way to cope with racism, sexism, transphobia, discrimination, violence, and a myriad of other oppressive/harmful levers and applications of systems. Identifying adaptive mistrust and critical evaluation of others, groups, or institutions of power is central to providing culturally sensitive and humble care.

## Microfiction

### 1,312 Days

Everyone leaves. They all leave. And by the same token, so do I. My life has been marked by cycles of comings and goings. No one ever advertises that their plan is to leave. The reasons, excuses, good-byes, and departures are always thoughtfully and carefully crafted. They're delicate in the choosing of words. They "break it" gently, with whispered tones,

DOI: 10.4324/9781003145943-4

gentle eyebrows, well-reasoned logic, and a series of explanations. I hear the undertones and urgent unstated wishes. "You understand, don't you? You agree, right, that this is best for everyone?"

I nod. I always nod. What did I expect? I believed them once, when they told me that I would be a part of their family. I believed then when they told me that I was important to them, when they made me feel as if my presence was required, in order for our family to be complete. I stopped believing them when the words stopped matching and I found myself packed again, so I nod.

I cross off another day in the notebook that is usually tucked into my bag. The scratching is a sound I recognize. This sound is consistent and familiar. Here we are: 1,312 until I turn 18. I have 1,312 days until I age out of foster care. I have 1,312 days until I leave.

*(Español)*

 **Microficción**

### *1,312 Dias*

*Todos se van. Todos se van. Y de la misma manera, yo también. Mi vida ha estado marcada por ciclos de idas y venidas. Nadie anuncia que su plan es irse. Las razones, excusas, despedidas y salidas siempre se elaboran concienzuda y cuidadosamente. Son delicados en la elección de palabras. Lo "rompen" suavemente, con tonos susurrados, cejas suaves, lógica bien razonada y una serie de explicaciones. Escucho los matices y los deseos urgentes no expresados. "Lo entiendes, ¿no es así? ¿Estás de acuerdo, verdad, en que esto es lo mejor para todos? "*

*Asiento con la cabeza. Yo siempre asiento con la cabeza. ¿Qué esperaba? Una vez les creí, cuando me dijeron que sería parte de su familia. Creí entonces cuando me dijeron que yo era importante para ellos, cuando me hicieron sentir que mi presencia era necesaria para que nuestra familia fuera completa. Dejé de creerles cuando las palabras dejaron de coincidir y me encontré empacado de nuevo, así que asentí.*

*Tacho otro día en el cuaderno que normalmente llevo metido en mi bolso. El rascado es un sonido que reconozco. Este sonido es consistente y familiar. Aquí estamos: 1,312 hasta que cumpla 18 años. Tengo 1,312 días hasta que salga de la crianza temporal. Tengo 1,312 días hasta que me vaya.*

Author: Noelany Pelc.

 **Processing questions for the clients (Preguntas de proceso para los/as clientes)**

1. In this story, we know so little about the main character's context, identities, and life outside of their thoughts in a brief moment in time. Even with this knowledge, what theme(s) permeate their inner dialogue? What thoughts and feelings bubble to the surface for you? (*En esta historia, sabemos muy poco sobre el contexto, las identidades y la vida del personaje principal fuera de sus pensamientos en un breve momento. Incluso con este conocimiento, ¿qué tema (s) impregnan su diálogo interno? ¿Qué pensamientos y sentimientos salen a la superficie para ti?*)

2. When have you felt like this character? In what ways have you all shared this moment? Discuss. (*¿Cuándo te has sentido como este personaje? ¿De qué manera habéis compartido todos este momento? Discutir.*)

3. How do you anticipate that they will engage with the world around them? How do you anticipate that they feel when they meet new individuals, make plans, consider long-term goals, and feel about themselves? Can you relate to any of these patterns? (*¿Cómo anticipa que se involucrarán con el mundo que los rodea? ¿Cómo anticipa que se sentirán cuando conozcan a nuevas personas, hagan planes, consideren metas a largo plazo y se sientan consigo mismos? ¿Puede identificarse con alguno de estos patrones?*)

4. "What if" their circumstances changed drastically tomorrow. How would they know? How long would it take them to believe that their life is different, and that they could trust the words that others share with them? (*"¿Y si?" Sus circunstancias cambiaran drásticamente mañana. ¿Cómo lo sabrían? ¿Cuánto tiempo les tomaría creer que su vida es diferente y que pueden confiar en las palabras que otros comparten con ellos?*)

5. What adaptive skills might this individual have learned, that will serve them in the future? On the contrary, what harmful messages might they be carrying with them that will limit their quality of life? Discuss. (*¿Qué habilidades de adaptación podría haber aprendido este individuo que le sirvan en el futuro? Por el contrario, ¿qué mensajes dañinos pueden llevar consigo que limitarán su calidad de vida? Discutir.*)

## Sayings (*dichos*)

### Saying #1

"It is an equal failing to trust everybody, and to trust nobody."
   "*Es una falla comparable no confiar en todos, y no confiar en nadie.*"

Author: Unknown. Popular English Proverb (Wood, 2019).

## Processing questions for the clients (Preguntas de proceso para los/as clientes)

1. Trusting or distrusting others often comes with limits, specifications, considerations, and past experiences, yet the rules of trust are easy to apply bluntly. What rules of trust do you apply to others? (*Confiar o desconfiar de los demás a menudo viene con límites, especificaciones, consideraciones y experiencias pasadas, sin embargo, las reglas de la confianza son fáciles de aplicar sin rodeos. ¿Qué reglas de confianza aplicas a los demás?*)

2. What is the central lesson of this saying? How do you enact this dilemma in your own life? (*¿Cuál es la lección central de este dicho? ¿Cómo representa este dilema en su propia vida?*)

3. Look at the image that follows. (*Mira la imagen de abajo.*)

   a. What comes to mind for you? (*¿Qué te viene a la mente?*)
   b. Which character would you be? (*¿Qué personaje serías tú?*)
   c. What do you think that they are thinking and feeling? How does this event end? (*¿Qué crees que están pensando y sintiendo? ¿Cómo termina este evento?*)

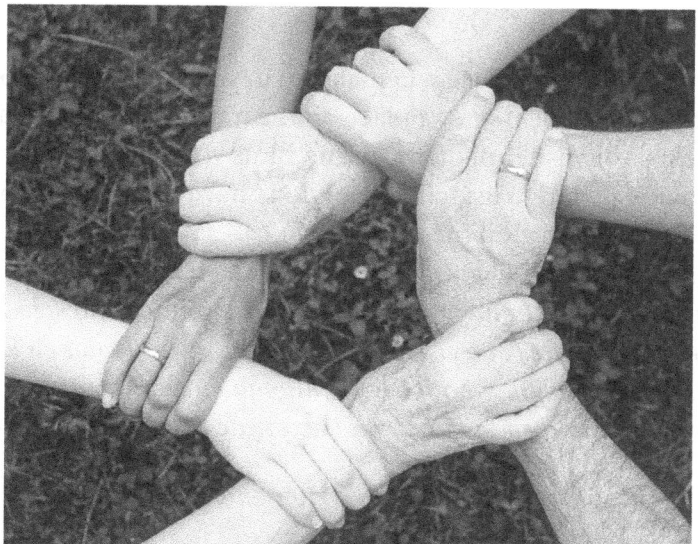

*Figure 2.1* Trusting in Others

### Saying #2

"When there is no enemy within you, the enemies outside cannot hurt you."
    *"Cuando no hay enemigo dentaro de ti, los enemigos de afuera no pueden lastimarte."*

Author: African Proverb (Stone, 2006).

### Processing questions for the clients (Preguntas de proceso para los/as clientes)

1. In what ways does this saying relate to trust? (*¿De qué manera se relaciona este dicho con la confianza?*)
2. How would you describe your most common enemies, both within and outside? (*¿Cómo describiría a sus enemigos más comunes, tanto dentro como fuera?*)
3. How would peace between your inner enemies change your life story? (*¿Cómo cambiaría la historia de su vida la paz entre sus enemigos internos?*)

## Quotes

### Quote #1a

"She might be without country, without nation, but inside her there was still a being that could exist and be free, that could simply say I am without adding a this, or a that, without saying I am Indian, Guyanese, English, or anything else in the world."
    *"Ella podría estar sin patria, sin nación, pero dentro de ella todavía había un ser que podía existir y ser libre, que podía simplemente decir yo soy sin agregar un esto, o aquello, sin decir que soy indio, guyanés, inglés, o cualquier otra cosa en el mundo."*

Author: Sharon Maas, author of *Of Marriageable Age* (2014), is a Guyanese-born novelist.

## Quote #1b

"Maybe your country is only a place you make up in your own mind. Something you dream about and sing about. Maybe it's not a place on the map at all, but just a story full of people you meet and places you visit, full of books and films you've been to. I'm not afraid of being homesick and having no language to live in. I don't have to be like anyone else. I'm walking on the wall and nobody can stop me."

*"Tal vez su país sea solo un lugar que usted crea en su propia mente. Algo con lo que sueñas y cantas. Tal vez no sea un lugar en el mapa en absoluto, sino solo una historia llena de personas que conoces y lugares que visitas, llena de libros y películas en las que has estado. No tengo miedo de sentir nostalgia y no tener un idioma en el que vivir. No tengo que ser como los demás. Estoy caminando en la pared y nadie puede detenerme."*

Author: Hugo Hamilton is a German-Irish writer and author of *The Speckled People* (2004).

## Processing questions for the clients (Preguntas de proceso para los/as clientes)

1. Read through both quotes and note your immediate reactions. To which quote do you most gravitate? Explain. (*Lea ambas citas y observe sus reacciones inmediatas. ¿A qué cita gravitas más? Explicar.*)
2. What shared elements do both quotes hold? Are there meaningful differences between them? (*¿Qué elementos compartidos contienen ambas citas? ¿Existen diferencias significativas entre ellos?*)
3. Are there elements that have led to you being "without country . . ." or nation, either through legal or political reasons, or as a result of more felt experiences? Discuss. (*¿Hay elementos que te hayan llevado a estar "sin país . . . " o nación, ya sea por razones legales o políticas, o como resultado de experiencias más sentidas? Discutir.*)
4. How do you describe your own relationship with your geographic home, ethnic roots, cultural ties, and familial home? Discuss how your own story is similar or different to what has been conveyed, and why. (*¿Cómo describe su propia relación con su hogar geográfico, raíces étnicas, vínculos culturales y hogar familiar? Discuta en qué se parece o difiere su propia historia de lo que se ha transmitido y por qué.*)

## Quote #2

"Have enough courage to trust love one more time and always one more time."
*"Ten el coraje suficiente para confiar en el amor una vez más y siempre una vez más."*

Author: Maya Angelou was an American poet and civil rights activist (Angelou, 2021).

## Processing questions for the clients (Preguntas de proceso para los/as clientes)

1. The author speaks of trusting love, although this quote can apply to trust in many scenarios, when interacting with others. How are courage and trust related, according to this quote? (*El autor habla de confiar en el amor, aunque esta cita puede aplicarse a la*

*confianza en muchos escenarios, al interactuar con los demás. ¿Cómo se relacionan el coraje y la confianza, según esta cita?)*

2. What are the interpersonal risks that require courage in relationships? (*¿Cuáles son los riesgos interpersonales que requieren valentía en las relaciones?*)

3. What can be gained by taking courageous interpersonal risks? (*¿Qué se puede ganar asumiendo valientes riesgos interpersonales?*)

4. Utilizing the link provided, scroll to the bottom of the page and complete the C.A.R.E. Relational Survey. Instructions for completing and interpreting your scores are provided. Discuss your findings and reflections on your relationships and patterns of trust. What recommended C.A.R.E. exercises can you complete to create movement toward more fulfilling and safe relationships? (*Utilizando el enlace proporcionado, desplácese hasta la parte inferior de la página y complete el C.A.R.E. Encuesta relacional. Se proporcionan instrucciones para completar e interpretar sus puntajes. Discuta sus hallazgos y reflexiones sobre sus relaciones y patrones de confianza. Lo que recomendó C.A.R.E. ejercicios que puede realizar para crear un movimiento hacia relaciones más satisfactorias y seguras?)*

Link: https://amybanksmd.com/about/#toggle-id-1

### Quote #3

"Trust only movement. Life happens at the level of events, not of words. Trust movement."
"*Confía solo en el movimiento. La vida pasa a nivel de eventos, no de palabras. Movimiento de confianza."*

Author: Alfred Adler was an Austrian physician and psychotherapist who founded the school of Individual Psychology (Adler, 2021).

### Processing questions for the clients (Preguntas de proceso para los/as clientes)

1. Imagine that your story were printed only as an illustrated book. This book holds no captions, text, explanations, or descriptors. What would someone flipping through these pages learn about you? (*Imagina que tu historia se imprimió sólo como un libro ilustrado. Este libro no contiene subtítulos, texto, explicaciones ni descriptores. ¿Qué aprendería sobre usted alguien que hojee estas páginas?)*

2. What dimensions are missing from this book, that would explain the choices, decisions, and actions that you take? Discuss comment bubbles, narrations, and internal dialogue that would offer context. (*¿Qué dimensiones faltan en este libro, que explicarían las elecciones, decisiones y acciones que toma? Discuta las burbujas de comentarios, las narraciones y el diálogo interno que ofrecerían contexto.)*

3. Select a moment in time that holds meaning for you. A moment that you believe has been pivotal for you, and which you wish you would have managed differently. Use the following format, and modify the structure as would be most helpful for you. Answer the following questions once you have completed the exercise: (*Seleccione un momento en el tiempo que tenga significado para usted. Un momento que crees que ha sido*

*fundamental para ti y que desearías haber manejado de otra manera. Utilice el siguiente formato y modifique la estructura como le resulte más útil. Responda las siguientes preguntas una vez que haya completado el ejercicio:)*

a. What do you know now, that was not available to you, then? (*¿Qué sabes ahora que no estaba disponible para ti, entonces?*)

b. What can you do to increase trust and coherence between your hopes for your character(s), and your actions, if anything? (*¿Qué puedes hacer para aumentar la confianza y la coherencia entre tus esperanzas para tu (s) personaje (s) y tus acciones, en todo caso?*)

Describe the event, in several lines. What happened leading up to the event, how did the event unfold, and what was the outcome? (*Describe el evento en varias líneas. ¿Qué sucedió antes del evento, cómo se desarrolló el evento y cuál fue el resultado?*)

_____

_____

_____

_____

_____

What characters were present? (*¿Qué personajes estuvieron presentes?*)

_____

_____

_____

_____

Illustrate the event on a piece of paper. Any art is welcome—abstract art and any tools or level of experience will be just as effective. (*Ilustre el evento en un pedazo de papel. Cualquier arte es bienvenido: el arte abstracto y cualquier herramienta o nivel de experiencia serán igualmente efectivos.*)

Offer narration. What would a narrator offer about what the primary character was thinking and feeling. Feel free to add comment bubbles or thought bubbles. (*Ofrezca la narración. ¿Qué ofrecería un narrador sobre lo que pensaba y sentía el personaje principal? Siéntase libre de agregar burbujas de comentarios o burbujas de pensamiento.*)

_____

_____

_____

_____

# References

Adler, A. (2021, March 3). www.quotes-clothing.com/trust-only-movement-life-happens-at-the-level-of-events-not-of-words-trust-movement-alfred-adler/

Angelou, M. (2021, June 12). www.goodreads.com/quotes/225830-have-enough-courage-to-trust-love-one-more-time-and

Hamilton, H. (2004). *The speckled people: A memoir of a half-Irish childhood.* HarperCollins.

Maas, S. (2014). *Of marriageable age.* Hachette Book Group.

Stone, J. R. (2006). *The Routledge book of world proverbs.* Taylor & Francis.

Wood, J. (2019). *Dictionary of quotations from ancient and modern, English and foreign sources.* Good Press.

# 3 Criticism

Human beings are influenced by an array of external forces that, when unfiltered, can cause more harm than good. In an era in which social media can establish trends and disseminate massive amounts of information in a matter of minutes, clients who have not developed a strong system of checks and balances to determine the veracity and quality of these sources are particularly vulnerable. Cultures, religions, societal trends, morals, values, and beliefs can be used as frameworks to justify non-constructive criticism. Untamed, non-constructive criticism can cause internal distress and psychological dysfunctions that ultimately affect the quality of life.

See also: forgiveness, humility and self-compassion, adversity, distress tolerance, and motivation

## Microfiction

### The Judge

A typical day. I browsed my phone and peeked at the news. A prominent celebrity is mocked because she gained weight after giving birth and suffering from postpartum depression. Another artist was body shamed after a paparazzi took unwanted pictures of him on a private beach. A politician was criticized and ultimately ostracized by the political party for making one incorrect statement. My daughter interrupts my "informative" reading by asking for a signature on a graded assignment. I smirked and told her: "Is B- your best effort? I guess that you should get off your phone and hit the books occasionally. If you want to be mediocre, continue this path." Ashamed, my daughter stormed to her bedroom and slammed the door. I checked the mail and noticed a past due notice from the electric/gas company. Irritated, I yelled at my wife: "How come you didn't pay this bill on time? It is not that we don't have the money to pay it, you should be ashamed of yourself. I only give you one responsibility and you cannot take care of it, then you ask me why I badmouth you. I guess that I am the only one in this house that has it together!"

*(Español)*

DOI: 10.4324/9781003145943-5

**Microficción**

*El Juez*

*Un día típico. Hojeé mi teléfono y eché un vistazo a las noticias. Se burla de una celebridad prominente porque ganó peso después de dar a luz y sufrir de depresión posparto. A otro artista se le avergonzó de su cuerpo después de que un paparazzi le tomó fotos no deseadas en una playa privada. Un político fue criticado y finalmente condenado al ostracismo por el partido político y por hacer una declaración incorrecta. Mi hija interrumpe mi lectura "informativa" al pedir una firma en una tarea calificada. Sonreí y le dije: "¿Cuál es tu mejor esfuerzo? Supongo que deberías quitarte el teléfono y leer los libros de vez en cuando. Si quieres ser mediocre, sigue ese camino". Avergonzada, mi hija irrumpió en su habitación y cerró la puerta. Revisé el correo y noté un aviso vencido de la compañía de electricidad/gas. Irritado, le grité a mi esposa: "¿Cómo es que no pagaste esta factura a tiempo? No es que no tengamos el dinero para pagarlo, debes avergonzarte de ti misma. Solo te doy una responsabilidad y no puedes ocuparte de ella, entonces me preguntas por qué te critico. ¡Supongo que soy el único en esta casa que lo tiene todo bajo control, caramba!"*
Author: Roberto Swazo.

 **Processing questions for the clients (Preguntas de proceso para los/as clientes)**

1. What seems to be the prevalent theme of this microfiction? (*¿Cuál parece ser el tema predominante de esta microficción?*)
2. Provide a list of three distinctive events in your life in which you were criticized by someone. How did you handle it? (*Proporciona una lista de tres eventos distintivos en tu vida en los que fuiste criticado por alguien. ¿Cómo lo manejaste?*)
3. What coping strategies do you have in order to distinguish between constructive versus destructive criticism? (*¿Qué estrategias de manejo tienes para distinguir entre la crítica constructiva y la crítica destructiva?*)
4. Which character in this story resembles you the most? Explain. (*¿Qué personaje de esta historia se parece más a ti? Explique.*)

*Cultural Hints*

Criticism might be an ingrained element for some cultures that use it to "motivate" others (typically children and family members) to achieve. The caveat is that not every individual person is willing to be constantly criticized, and that applies to members of cultures in which this is an acceptable practice. So, as a practitioner, one has to validate the utilization of criticism as a motivational tool from a cultural standpoint while acknowledging the unique subjective experience of the client. In many ways and as a common practice a cultural practice that feels oppressive and is causing emotional turmoil to a client needs to be evaluated from a "cultural criticism" standpoint. Keep in mind that not all cultural practices are healthy and beneficial to its members as they transcend cultural tolerance by entering the realm of universal human rights (i.e., female genital mutilation, literacy bans against girls, etc.).

·)) 🎧 **Sayings (*dichos*)**

### *Saying #1*

"When ignorance envies and criticizes, intelligence observes, listens and laughs."
"*Cuando la ignorancia envidia y critica, la inteligencia observa, escucha y se ríe.*"

Author: Unknown. Latin American saying (F. Ramirez, personal communication, April 11, 2018).

·)) 🎧 **Processing questions for the clients (Preguntas de proceso para los/as clientes)**

1. Browse the Internet, news, and other social media and pinpoint how many news, opinions, and analyses are based on criticism. What does it say about our current societal environment? Explain. (*Explora la Internet, noticias y otras redes sociales y señala cuántas noticias, opiniones y análisis se basan en las críticas. ¿Qué dice esto sobre nuestro entorno social actual? Explique.*)
2. Do you have the capacity to laugh at yourself when you make a mistake? Elaborate. (*¿Tienes la capacidad de reírte de ti mismo cuando cometes un error? Elabora.*)
3. From your favorite movies, which character would you like to be or at least emulate? What are their prominent traits? What does it say about you at this moment? (*De tus películas favoritas, ¿qué personaje te gustaría ser o al menos emular? ¿Cuáles son sus rasgos prominentes?¿Qué dice esto de ti en estos momentos?*)

·)) 🎧 ### *Saying #2*

"The wound caused by a spear can heal, but that caused by the tongue is incurable."
"*La herida causada por una lanza puede curar, pero la causada por la lengua es incurable.*"

Author: Unknown. Arabic proverb (S. Assad, personal communication, April 11, 2018).

·)) 🎧 **Processing questions for the clients (Preguntas de proceso para los/as clientes)**

1. How many times have you been hurt by words? What specifically hurts you the most when it is said about you? (*¿Cuántas veces has sido lastimado por las palabras? ¿Qué es lo que más te duele específicamente cuando se habla de ti?*)
2. It is possible that things said about you are right and yet, they still hurt you. Do you have the ability to engage in an honest process of self-evaluation? List the aspects that you are often criticized about—do you see a trend? (*Es posible que las cosas que se dicen sobre ti sean correctas y, sin embargo, aún te lastiman. ¿Tienes la capacidad de envolverte en un proceso honesto de autoevaluación? Haz una lista de los aspectos por los cuales se te critican a menudo, ¿ves una tendencia?*)
3. Draw a picture of an emotional wound. Describe its depth, sensitivity, pain, etc. (*Haz un dibujo de una herida emocional. Descríbelo. Profundidad, sensibilidad, dolor, etc.*)
4. Take your family picture and identify those family members who are critical of others. Have you found yourself repeating some family behavioral patterns? Elaborate. (*Toma*

*una fotografía de tu familia e identifica a los miembros de tu familia que critican a los demás. ¿Te has encontrado repitiendo algunos patrones de comportamiento de tu familia? Elabore.)*

## Quotes

 *Quote #1*

"It is much valuable to look for the strengths in others. You can gain nothing by criticizing their imperfections."

*"Es mucho más valioso buscar las fortalezas en los demás. No puedes ganar nada criticando sus imperfecciones."*

Author: Daisaku Ikeda. He is a Japanese Buddhist philosopher, educator, author, and nuclear disarmament advocate (2013).

**Processing questions for the clients (Preguntas de proceso para los/as clientes)**

1. Engage in a serious self-assessment process by doing the following: (*Participa en un proceso serio de autoevaluación haciendo lo siguiente:*)

   a. Read the news and immediately register your gut reactions about celebrities, politicians, or those who are writing the news. (*Lee las noticias e inmediatamente registra tus reacciones viscerales sobre celebridades, políticos o aquellos que están escribiendo las noticias.*)

   b. At large, how are these reactions? Negative or positive? Explain. How much cynicism and negativism do they contain? (*En general, ¿cómo son estas reacciones? ¿Negativas o positivas? ¿Cuánto cinismo y negativismo contienen? Explica.*)

2. When you look at your coworkers, friends, neighbors, community members, and relatives, do you look for their imperfections and negative attributes? Or, do you praise their positive attributes? (*Cuando observas a tus compañeros de trabajo, amigos, vecinos, miembros de la comunidad y parientes, ¿buscas sus imperfecciones y atributos negativos? ¿O elogias tus atributos positivos?*)

3. **Homework assignment:** Every day for two weeks you will select one person (i.e., friend, relative, coworker, politician, etc.) and make a list of positive traits about them. Concentrate only on the positive attributes. Then, select at least five to seven people and tell them that you admire and commend them for having these attributes. Register how you feel about doing this. How does it change your perception of people in general? Repeat this exercise mentally on a daily basis and if you have the opportunity, and praise the individual on the spot.

   (*Asignación: Todos los días durante dos semanas seleccionarás a una persona (es decir, amigo, pariente, compañero de trabajo, político, etc.) y harás una lista de rasgos positivos sobre él/ella. Concéntrate sólo en los atributos positivos. Luego, selecciona al menos cinco a siete personas y díles que los admiras y felicitas por tener estos atributos. Registra cómo te sientes al hacer esto. ¿Cómo cambia tu percepción de las personas en general? Repite este ejercicio mentalmente a diario y, si tienes la oportunidad, elogia al individuo en el acto.)*

## Quote #2

"If we are so given to judging others, it is because we tremble for ourselves."

"*Si nosotros somos tan dados a juzgar a los demás, es debido a que temblamos por nosotros mismos.*"

Author: Oscar Wilde. He was an Irish wit, poet, and dramatist (2021).

## Processing questions for the clients (Preguntas de proceso para los/as clientes)

1. What is your most immediate reaction when someone criticizes you? Elaborate. (*¿Cuál es tu reacción más inmediata cuando alguien te critica? Elaborar.*)
2. Do you think that all criticism about you is unfounded? Have you heard more than one person pointing out the same things to you? Do you have the innate reaction to retaliate by doing the same thing? (*¿Crees que todas las críticas sobre ti son infundadas? ¿Has escuchado a más de una persona que te señala las mismas cosas? ¿Tienes la reacción innata de tomar represalias haciéndoles lo mismo?*)
3. Do you take criticism as a personal attack or as an opportunity to grow, expand, and develop as a human being? What is your fear of feedback from others? (*¿Tomas tú las críticas como un ataque personal o como una oportunidad para crecer, expandirte y desarrollarte como ser humano? ¿Cuál es tu miedo a la retroalimentación de parte de otros?*)

## Quote #3

"Gossip is like smoke because it dissipates quickly, but it blackens everything it touches."

"*La murmuración se parece al humo porque se disipa pronto, pero ennegrece todo lo que toca.*"

Author: Madame De Staël. She was a Franco-Swiss woman of letters and political theorist of Genevan origin (2021).

## *Cultural Hints*

In some cultures, gossip is part of lifestyle and widely accepted as a way of communication. On the other hand, "cultural acceptance" does not mean that a person has to condone it and live by its cannons. This is especially true if the person has to operate in another culture where this is not accepted and might be detrimental to their career, sense of self, and relationships. As a result, the client might have to navigate two different sets of cultures by using cultural code switching or by simply disowning gossip as a communication strategy in order to preserve their emotional integrity.

**Processing questions for the clients (Preguntas de proceso para los/as clientes)**

1. Take a glass of milk and drop by drop start adding chocolate to it. Stir it up each time and look at the effect. Compare it to another glass of milk without the drops of chocolate. Not only are there changes of color but the flavor of milk is altered as well. How many drops of gossip do you add to the lives of others on a daily basis? How many of these drops are being added to your life by others? What can you do about this? Explain. (*Toma un vaso de leche y gota a gota comienza a agregarle chocolate. Revuelve todo el tiempo y mira el efecto. Compáralo con otro vaso de leche sin las gotas de chocolate. No solo hay cambios de color, sino que también se altera el sabor de la leche. ¿Cuántas gotas de chismes agregas a la vida de los demás a diario? ¿Cuántas de estas gotas están siendo agregadas a tu vida por otros? ¿Qué puedes hacer al respecto? Explica.*)

2. **Homework:** Go to a partner, friend, coworker, or relative and nonchalantly make a positive comment about somebody else. This is an antidote to gossip as it does not contaminate but nurses the environment and your emotional well. Evaluate yourself and the reactions of others. (*Tarea: ve donde un/a socio/a, amigo/a, compañero/a de trabajo o pariente y haz un comentario positivo sobre otra persona. Este es un antídoto contra los chismes, ya que no contamina pero cuida el medio ambiente y tu bienestar emocional. Evalúate a ti mismo y a las reacciones de los demás.*)

3. If you gossip about others, what purpose does it serve for you? Are you overcompensating for an emotional, physical, or psychological need? What are these? Do you have the willingness to identify them by name? (*Si chismeas sobre otros, ¿para qué te sirve? ¿Estás sobrecompensando una necesidad emocional, física o psicológica? ¿Cuáles son estas? ¿Tienes la voluntad de identificarlas por su nombre?*)

## References

De Staël, M. (2021, October 27). www.inspiringquotes.us/author/4492-madame-de-stael

Ikeda, D. (2013). *Discussions on youth: For the leaders of the future.* Middleway Press.

Wilde, O. (2021, January 24). www.brainyquote.com/authors/oscar-wilde-quotes

# 4 Forgiveness

Forgiveness is at the core of human healing. Non-forgiveness or holding a grudge can be equated to a festering infection that consumes a person inside out during a long and painful process. Forgiveness takes on many forms, and it is one of the most prevalent themes in any therapeutic setting. For instance, some clients have a hard time forgiving themselves for events that occurred many years ago. They are tormented by non-stop and intrusive thoughts that act like a corroding cancer. Likewise, other clients have a hard time forgiving parents, siblings, or friends for words said or actions that seem unforgivable. Similarly, other clients are angry at life, social and religious organizations, or political parties, others cannot forgive G-d or a creator for things that have happened to them. How do people who survived the European Holocaust forgive their Nazi perpetrators? Where do some individuals muster the strength to forgive a criminal who murdered a child or a spouse? Forgiveness can be defined as one of the most powerful healing tools in order to experience liberation, growth, and a fruitful life in the absence of an emotional illness.

See also: relationships, change, future, and hope

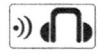 ## Microfiction

### *The Golden Coins*

There was a small orphanage in Spain dedicated to the rescue of children who were victims of war, many of whom were absorbed as the result of the Holocaust. This particular orphanage was devoted to rescuing girls who had lost their parents and whose relatives were untraceable. A Sephardic Jewish philanthropic woman who herself came from an orphanage but had managed to get an education and create a buoyant import and export line of textiles from North Africa dedicated all her free time to the orphanage and to giving an opportunity to these orphans. One day, she came to visit the orphanage with the purpose of monitoring the facilities and getting to know some of the new girls who were rescued and placed in the building. As usual, she placed her purse on top of a cabinet and proceeded to spend time walking around, conversing with the girls, and some of the people in charge of this particular shift. When she was ready to take off, she noticed that her purse was open and some golden coins were missing. She talked to some of the staff about the situation, and they felt ashamed about it. Some staff wanted to conduct a thorough search and find the girl who stole the golden coins and reprimand her heavily. Various staff members were enraged and could not understand how anyone would do something like

DOI: 10.4324/9781003145943-6

that to the person who provided shelter, meals, medical service, protection, education, and a future. However, the philanthropic woman had a plan that baffled everyone. She ordered the staff to leave the area where the girls were and close the doors behind. She stayed in the room alone with the girls and told them to stand facing their beds. Then, she ordered all of them to close their eyes and instructed whoever had the golden coins to throw them over their shoulders to the center of the room. Suddenly, the clicking sound of the golden coins reverberated the sordid and deafening silence. The philanthropic woman proceeded to turn around and had them open their eyes. They saw that the coins were sitting on the floor. Suddenly, an accusing voice from one of the girls yelled: "Who was it? Who was so ungrateful to steal from you who has been so good to us?" Then, the philanthropic woman paused and said: "I don't know either; I didn't see anything, I also had my eyes closed. Everything has been forgiven. Nobody has been shamed."

(*Español*)

 **Microficción**

### Las Monedas de Oro

*Había un pequeño orfanato en España dedicado al rescate de niños víctimas de la guerra muchos de los cuales fueron absorbidos como consecuencia del holocausto. Este orfanato en particular se dedicó a rescatar a niñas que perdieron a sus padres y cuyos familiares no pudieron rastrear. Una mujer filantrópica judía sefardí la cual se había criado en un orfanato pero que había logrado obtener una educación y crear una línea boyante de importación y exportación de textiles del norte de África, dedicó todo su tiempo libre al orfanato y a dar una oportunidad a estos huérfanos. Un día, vino a visitar el orfanato con el propósito de monitorear las instalaciones y conocer a algunas de las nuevas niñas que fueron rescatadas y colocadas en el edificio. Como de costumbre, colocó su bolso encima de un gabinete y pasó un tiempo caminando, conversando con las chicas y algunas de las personas a cargo de este turno en particular. Cuando estuvo lista para salir, notó que su bolso estaba abierto y faltaban algunas monedas de oro. Habló con algunos miembros del personal sobre la situación los cuales se sintieron avergonzados por la misma. Algunos miembros del personal querían realizar una búsqueda exhaustiva y encontrar a la niña que había robado las monedas de oro y reprender duramente. Varios miembros del personal estaban enfurecidos y no podían entender cómo alguien podría hacerle algo así a la persona que le proporcionó refugio, comida, servicio médico, protección, educación y un futuro. Sin embargo, la mujer filantrópica tenía un plan que desconcertó a todos. Ella ordenó al personal que abandonara el área donde estaban las niñas y que cerraran las puertas al momento de salir. Se quedó en la habitación sola con las niñas y les dijo que se pararan frente a sus camas. Así, les ordenó a todas que cerraran los ojos e instruyó a quien tuviera las monedas de oro que las arrojara sobre sus hombros hacia el centro de la habitación. De repente, el chasquido de las monedas de oro reverberaba en el sórdido y ensordecer silencio. La filantrópica les hizo dar la vuelta y abrir los ojos. Vieron que las monedas estaban en el suelo. De repente, una voz acusadora de una de las niñas gritó: "¿Quién fue? ¿Quién fue tan ingrata para robarle a la que ha sido tan buena con nosotros? Entonces, la mujer filantrópica hizo una pausa y dijo: "Yo tampoco lo sé; No vi nada, también tenía los ojos cerrados. Todo ha sido perdonado. Nadie ha sido avergonzada."*
Author: Roberto Swazo.

*Cultural Hints*

Forgiveness has been typically associated with religion in Western cultures, however, it is a universal theme that transcends countries, languages, and philosophies. The concept of shame can be devastating in Asian cultures while in Western cultures it has been primarily used as a punishment mechanism. Shame can also be destructive and a major producer of lifelong emotional scars.

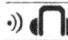 **Processing questions for the clients (Preguntas de proceso para los/as clientes)**

1.  After reading the story, take a notebook or a piece of paper and write down an emotional summary of the story. That is, what are the key emotional reactions that you could extract from this story? Explain. (*Después de leer la historia, tome un cuaderno o una hoja de papel y escriba un resumen emocional de la historia. Es decir, ¿cuáles son las reacciones emocionales clave que podrías extraer de esta historia? Explicar.*)

2.  It sounds like the philanthropic woman had gone through very difficult times in her life and yet, she decided to devote part of her life to this orphanage and the children. Obviously, she had the means to have a rich and plentiful life in which she could spend her money in extravagant luxuries but decided not to only do this. Why? Elaborate. (*Parece que la mujer filantrópica había pasado por momentos muy difíciles en su vida y, sin embargo, decidió dedicar parte de su vida a este orfanato ya los niños. Obviamente, tenía los medios para tener una vida rica y abundante en la que podía gastar su dinero en lujos extravagantes, pero decidió no solo hacer esto. ¿Por qué? Elaborar.*)

3.  Why do you think that the philanthropic woman decided to close her eyes and not look at the girl who stole the golden coins? Discuss. (*¿Por qué crees que la dama filantrópica decidió cerrar los ojos y no mirar a la niña que robó las monedas de oro? Discutir.*)

4.  If you would have been her, today, what would have been your reaction to being stolen from and do you think that you would have been able to forgive the girl who did it? Explain. (*Si hoy hubieras sido ella, ¿cuál habría sido tu reacción ante el robo y crees que habrías podido perdonar a la chica que lo hizo? Explicar.*)

 **Sayings (*dichos*)**

 *Sayings #1ab*

1a. "If there were no wrongdoing, there would be no forgiveness."
    "*Si no hubiera nada malo, no habría perdón.*"

   Author: Egyptian Proverb (Proverbicals.com, 2021).

1b. "If you offend, ask for pardon; if offended, forgive."
    "*Si ofendes, pide perdón; si te ofenden, perdona.*"

   Author: Ethiopian Proverb (African Proverbs, 2021).

 **Processing questions for the clients (Preguntas de proceso para los/as clientes)**

1.  What does quote (a) say about the nature of human beings? Explain.

   (*¿Qué dice la cita sobre la naturaleza de los seres humanos? Explicar.*)

2. Based on quote (a), how many times have you felt that others make mistakes that are unforgivable but your mistakes are minimal and easy to dismiss? Discuss.

   (*Según la cita (a), ¿cuántas veces has sentido que otros cometen errores imperdonables, pero tus errores son mínimos y fáciles de descartar? Discutir.*)

3. Based on quote (b) what is easier for you, to ask for an apology or to let go of emotional grudges? Can you cite examples from your daily life activities?

   (*Según la cita (b), ¿qué es más fácil para ti, pedir disculpas o dejar ir los rencores emocionales? ¿Puedes citar ejemplos de tus actividades de la vida diaria?*)

### Sayings #2ab

2a. "Forgiveness is a pillar of justice."
   "*El perdón es un pilar de la justicia.*"

   Author: Russian Proverb (Kalimaquotes.com, 2021).

2b. "Forgiveness is more satisfying than revenge."
   "*El perdón es más satisfactorio que la venganza.*"

   Author: Arabian Proverb (Idlehearts.com, 2021).

### Processing questions for the clients (Preguntas de proceso para los/as clientes)

1. What does it mean that forgiveness is a pillar of justice? Perhaps you might have to provide a personal definition of justice in order to provide a more substantive answer. (*¿Qué significa que el perdón es un pilar de la justicia? Quizás debas proporcionar una definición personal de justicia para poder dar una respuesta más sustantiva.*)

2. Based on quote (b), how can forgiving someone be more satisfying than exercising revenge? Explain. (*Según la cita (b), ¿cómo puede ser más satisfactorio perdonar a alguien que ejercer la venganza? Explicar.*)

3. Create a relaxation environment that allows you to transport yourself to a place, time, and specific event with other people that triggers an extremely negative emotion and the instinct to retaliate and get vengeance. Recreate this scenario and imagine yourself speaking to them calmly, empathically, and in a courteous way. Look them in the eye and clearly tell them that you forgive them. Then, walk away. This is a powerful scenario. Break down your emotions.

   (*Crea un ambiente de relajación que te permite transportarte a un lugar, tiempo y evento específico con otras personas que desencadenan una emoción extremadamente negativa y el instinto de tomar represalias y vengarse. Recrea este escenario e imagínate hablándoles con calma, empatía y cortesía. Míralos a los ojos y diles claramente que los perdonas. Luego, aléjate. Este es un escenario poderoso. Desglosa tus emociones.*)

### Quotes

### Quote #1

"Always forgive your enemies—nothing annoys them so much."
   "*Siempre perdona a tus enemigos—nada les molesta tanto.*"

Author: Oscar Wilde. He was an Irish poet and dramatist who was a spokesman for the late 19th-century Aesthetic movement that advocated for the love of art (2017).

**Processing questions for the clients (Preguntas de proceso para los/as clientes)**

1. Have you ever received forgiveness in your life knowing that you had made a mistake and you were wrong? Provide details. (*¿Alguna vez has recibido el perdón en tu vida sabiendo que habías cometido un error y estabas equivocado? Proporcionar detalles.*)
2. Imagine that one day you receive a letter that reads: "ALL your loans, including mortgage, personal, student, car, and credit cards have been forgiven. You are free of debt. A good hearted person decided to pay them for you. You do not owe one cent to anyone." Imagine! What questions would you ask? What would you do from now on? In what way would you repay this favor, as you do not know the person or institution that paid it all? Describe this process. (*Imagínate que un día recibes una carta que dice: "TODOS sus préstamos, incluidos los hipotecarios, personales, de estudiante, de automóvil y de crédito, han sido perdonados. Estás libre de deudas. Una persona de buen corazón decidió pagarlas por ti. No le debes ni un centavo a nadie". ¡Imagina! ¿Qué preguntas harías? ¿Qué harías a partir de ahora? ¿De qué manera pagarías este favor sin saber que no conoces a la persona o institución que lo pagó todo? Describe este proceso.*)

*Quote #2*

"To forgive is to set a prisoner free and discover that the prisoner was you."
   "*Perdonar es liberar a un prisionero y descubrir que el prisionero eras tú.*"

Author: Louis B. Smedes. He was a renowned Christian author, ethicist, and theologian in the Reformed tradition. He served as a professor of theology and ethics at Fuller Theological Seminary in Pasadena, California (2007).

**Processing questions for the clients (Preguntas de proceso para los/as clientes)**

1. Describe the picture that follows. What comes to your mind? (*Describe la imagen de abajo. ¿Qué te viene a la mente?*)

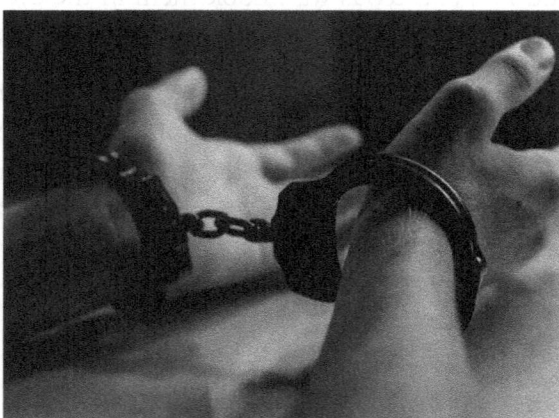

*Figure 4.1* A Person's Hands in Handcuffs

2. If one is a prisoner, then one is devoid of freedom. According to the quote, if one forgives freedom is achieved. Explain. (*Si uno es un prisionero, entonces está desprovisto de libertad. Según la cita, si uno perdona se logra la libertad. Explicar.*)

3. Make a list of the people, things, religious organizations, political groups, and family members that you are unable to forgive. Devise a plan on how to forgive these, step by step and try to execute these micro plans in a staggered way. (*Haz una lista de las personas, cosas, organizaciones religiosas, grupos políticos y miembros de la familia que no puedes perdonar. Diseña un plan sobre cómo perdonarlos, paso a paso, e intenta ejecutar estos micro planes de manera escalonada.*)

*Table 4.1* Three Columns Labeled, "Things," "Memories," and "Plan on How to Forgive Them." Four Intersecting Rows Labeled, "Events," "Religious Organizations," "Political Groups," and "Family Members."

| Things (Cosas ) | Memories (Recuerdos ) | Plan on how to forgive them (Plan de cómo perdonarles ) |
|---|---|---|
| Events (Eventos) | | |
| Religious organizations (Organizaciones religiosas) | | |
| Political groups (Grupos políticos) | | |
| Family members (Miembros de familia) | | |

### Quote #3

"The weak can never forgive. Forgiveness is the attribute of the strong."
"*Los débiles nunca pueden perdonar. El perdón es el atributo de los fuertes.*"

Author: Mahatma Gandhi. He was an Indian lawyer, politician, social activist, and writer who became the leader of the nationalist movement against the British rule of India (1990).

### Processing questions for the clients (Preguntas de proceso para los/as clientes)

1. How is it possible that forgiveness is a sign of strength? Are you able to picture this in your life? If so, under what circumstances? (*¿Cómo es posible que el perdón sea un signo de fuerza? ¿Puedes imaginar esto en tu vida? De ser así, ¿bajo qué circunstancias?*)

2. One way to move on with your life leaving behind anger and hate is by short-circuiting the cognitive and emotional rumination. For instance, how much time do you devote to negative thinking patterns associated with the person, institution, or event that is hurting you? As an exercise, be on the alert mode every time one of these memories comes to your mind and immediately stop these and conduct an *emotional replacement process*. Since the person/s or events are out of your control, you can control these related

emotions with positive emotions based on the future and immediate present. This does not mean that you are brushing these negative emotions under the rug but that you are simply experiencing the vestiges or leftovers of emotions and thoughts that have been solved. Doing this takes a hyper sense of awareness and self-control!

*(Una forma de seguir adelante con tu vida dejando atrás la ira y el odio es acortando la rumia cognitiva y emocional. Por ejemplo, ¿cuánto tiempo le dedicas a los patrones de pensamiento negativos asociados con la persona, institución o evento que te está lastimando? Como ejercicio, mantente alerta cada vez que uno de estos recuerdos te venga a la mente, detenlos inmediatamente y lleva a cabo un proceso de reemplazo emocional. Dado que las personas o los eventos están fuera de tu control, puedes controlar estas emociones relacionadas con emociones positivas basadas en el futuro y el presente inmediato. Esto no significa que estés enviando estas emociones negativas debajo de la alfombra, sino que simplemente estás experimentando los vestigios o restos de emociones y pensamientos que se han resuelto. ¡Hacer esto requiere un gran sentido de conciencia y autocontrol!)*

3.  Self-forgiveness will make you a stronger human being. Many times we can be our worst enemies by setting high moral standards that can never be achieved.

Still relatively unknown in North America, Naikan therapy is a Japanese practice of self-reflection that involves an arduous method of meditation. The traditional and most rigorous form of Naikan involves a degree of sensory deprivation and isolation and is practiced in Naikan centers for one week. You might not be able to attend a Naikan retreat, but you can start by focusing on the three questions:

a.  What have you received?
a.  What have you returned?
b.  What trouble have you caused?

4.  These three questions seek to achieve personal balance leading to self-forgiveness. Answer these questions on a daily basis in an attempt to refocus on the positive things that you have received and caused.

*(El perdonarte a ti mismo te hará un ser humano más fuerte. Muchas veces podemos ser nuestros peores enemigos si establecemos altos estándares morales que nunca podrán alcanzarse.*

*Aún relativamente desconocida en América del Norte, la terapia Naikan es una práctica japonesa de autorreflexión que implica un arduo método de meditación. La forma tradicional y más rigurosa de Naikan implica un grado de privación sensorial y aislamiento y se practica en los centros de Naikan durante una semana. Es posible que no pueda asistir a los retiros de Naikan, pero puedes comenzar concentrándote en las tres preguntas:*

a.  *¿Qué has recibido?*
b.  *¿Qué has devuelto?*
c.  *¿Qué problema has causado?*

*Estas tres preguntas buscan lograr un equilibrio personal que conduzca al perdón a uno mismo. Responde estas preguntas a diario y en un intento de volver a centrarte en las cosas positivas que has recibido y causado.)*

# References

African Proverbs. (2021, September 15). *Proverbs*. www.educationworld.com/a_tsl/TM/WS_african_ proverbs.shtml

Egyptian Proverbs. (2021, February 19). https://proverbicals.com/egyptian-proverbs

Gandhi, M. (1990). *All men are brothers: Autobiographical reflections*. Continuum.

Idlehearts (2021, July 23). www.idlehearts.com/328709/forgiveness-satisfying-revenge

Kalima Quotes. (2021, August 12). www.kalimaquotes.com/quotes/17619/forgiveness-is-a-pillar

Smedes, L. B. (2007). *Forgive and forget: Healing the hurts we don't deserve*. Harper Collins.

Wilde, O. (2017). *Oscar Wilde—a Florentine tragedy: Always forgive your enemies; nothing annoys them so much*. Stage Door.

# 5  Humility and Self-Compassion

Clinicians are intimately aware of the internal voices that clients discuss—the ways in which they talk with themselves; the expectations that they hold; the ways in which they motivate, challenge, chastise, and admonish themselves. Truly, this is a human experience that extends beyond the therapy room but that is often brought into therapy and is a central theme for many discussions and heartache.

*Humility*, in Western literature, is a relatively newer construct. There has been a shift away from striving to achieve high self-esteem, which involves comparing oneself and one's performance to that of others, and into a more human and *stable* self-esteem, which allows for more flexibility in managing challenges and achievements. At its core, humility allows for a more compassionate approach to acknowledging mistakes (which everyone is bound to make), to cultivating a more realistic and accurate sense of self, to being open to new perspectives, decreasing self-centeredness, and valuing the contributions of others. *Self-compassion* works in tandem with humility, and allows individuals to acknowledge their own suffering and pain, as a personal and human experience. This awareness allows clients to be mindful in the ways that they comfort and soothe themselves, and increases the likelihood of using more adaptive and effective coping strategies. Self-compassion, then, is centered around three main principles (Neff, 2021). The first of these is the understanding that all humans are imperfect and will at some point fall short. This allows individuals to be kind in their own internal dialogue and reduce shame. The second component involves shifting from a focus on suffering as an individual experience to a more universal and human experience. This perspective allows for a sense of universality and connectedness with others. Finally, self-compassion involves the acknowledgement and acceptance of thoughts and feelings, without becoming anchored to the emotional reactions that are attached to these feelings. Attending mindfully to responses allows individuals to hold them in balance, without overexaggerating their importance or impact.

Humility and self-compassion, then, are not only internal experiences, but also seep into relationships and interactions with others. Exploring the ways in which clients view themselves and manage obstacles, establish accurate views of themselves, and balance between pridefulness or ego and humility and self-compassion can be central to building a healthy relationship with themselves and those around them.

See also: relationships, criticism, and death and grief, and coping

DOI: 10.4324/9781003145943-7

## Cultural Hints

The definition and experience of humility can vary drastically depending on country of origin, cultural perspective, and level of identification with various identities. For some cultures in which family units or broader collectives take greater importance, discussions of self-compassion or balanced self-reflection may be a challenge. Framing discussions and explorations as opportunities to develop balance and humility in ways that are kind to the self and others may resonate more closely with personal and cultural values. Additionally, taking a *culturally humble* stance as mental health providers allows clinicians to model *not knowing*, recognizing limitations and gaps in understanding, and focusing on the other individual, particularly around the lived experiences across cultures.

## Microfiction

### The Touchstone

I squeeze my hand shut, a vice that restricts, more than protects. My fingers tremble from extended fatigue, and are mimicked by the muscles binding my hands, wrists, and forearm, as if they'll shake loose what I won't willingly produce. My breath lightens as I open my palm only enough to slide my thumb through the small gap. *Why do I even carry this?!* The thought is angry—shouted, almost.

"Paola! Let's go!" I whip my head, the movement simultaneously accompanied by a clenching of my hand. I slide my hand into the small pocket of my skirt. It stays with me, but out of sight. It always stays with me.

I hear my steps scuff the stony slats around the overhang. My friends are already gathered in a loose circle. Priti, James, Kwame, and Bennu are unpacking various bags, packages, and paper wrappers. My gaze slides over the ring, finding the spot that I always claim. The spot that belongs to me, without negotiation or words.

I curl my legs beneath me until I am in a squatted position and roughly wipe my damp hands on my skirt before my fingers find their way to the stone in my pocket. Already, my heart is skipping like it knows; tapping out a warning. The stone tumbles out, skittering under brambles as my arm flies out, as my fingers catch its familiar edge. I've found it for the second time, I realize, and smile softly. The first time I found it was on the beach at home, in my own country. It had wedged itself between my sandal and the hole I was digging, and something about its odd shape called to me. It stayed with me. It always stays with me.

I never share it, but I have decided that today is the day.

*And what if they don't like it?* I hear my own voice. *And what if they don't like its texture? What if they don't like its shape? What if they don't like its size? What if they miss the point? But it is me. It is all of me. It is a touchstone because it is a memory. It is my family, it is a piece of my roots. It is my land. It is my past, my present, and a wish for my future.*

"Paola! You're always late! We already put our treasures on the ground. Come on! What did you bring?"

My eyes snap up as I tip my head, and legs begin to uncoil. I cradle the stone in my open palm and pause. "I like it," I murmur quietly. "I like it."

My palm remains open as I move toward my circle of friends.

(*Español*)

## Microficción

### *La Piedra de Toque*

*Aprieto mi mano para cerrarla, un vicio que restringe, más que protege. Mis dedos tiemblan por la fatiga prolongada, e imitados por los músculos que sujetan mis manos, muñecas y antebrazo, como si fueran a soltar lo que no voy a producir voluntariamente. Mi respiración se aclara cuando abro la palma de mi mano solo lo suficiente para deslizar mi pulgar a través del pequeño espacio. ¡¿Por qué llevo esto?! El pensamiento es enfadado, casi gritado.*

*¡Paola! ¡Vamos!" Agito mi cabeza, el movimiento acompañado simultáneamente por un apretón de mi mano. Deslizo mi mano en el pequeño bolsillo de mi falda. Se queda conmigo, pero fuera de la vista. Siempre se queda conmigo.*

*Oigo que mis pasos raspan los listones de piedra que rodean el saliente. Mis amigos ya están reunidos en un círculo suelto, Priti, James, Kwame y Bennu están desempacando varias bolsas, paquetes y envoltorios de papel. Mi mirada se desliza sobre el anillo, encontrando el lugar que siempre reclamo. El lugar que me pertenece, sin negociación ni palabras.*

*Doblo mis piernas debajo de mí hasta que estoy en una posición en cuclillas y me limpio las manos húmedas en mi falda antes de que mis dedos encuentren el camino hacia la piedra en mi bolsillo. Ya, mi corazón está saltando como sabe; tocando una advertencia. La piedra cae, deslizándose bajo las zarzas mientras mi brazo sale volando, mientras mis dedos agarran su borde familiar. Lo he encontrado por segunda vez, me doy cuenta y sonrío suavemente. La primera vez que lo encontré fue en la playa de mi casa, en mi propio país. Se había encajado entre mi sandalia y el agujero que estaba cavando, y algo en su extraña forma me llamó la atención. Se quedó conmigo. Siempre se queda conmigo.*

*Nunca lo comparto, pero he decidido que hoy es el día.*

*¿Y si no les gusta? Escucho mi propia voz. ¿Y si no les gusta su textura? ¿Y si no les gusta su forma? ¿Qué pasa si no les gusta su tamaño? ¿Y si pierden el punto? Pero soy yo. Es todo de mí.*

*Es una piedra de toque porque es un recuerdo. Es mi familia, es un pedazo de mis raíces. Es mi tierra. Es mi pasado, mi presente y un deseo para mi futuro.*

*¡Paola! ¡Siempre llegas tarde! Ya pusimos nuestros tesoros en el suelo. ¡Vamos! ¿Qué trajiste?*

*Mis ojos se levantan cuando inclino la cabeza y las piernas comienzan a desenrollarse. Sostengo la piedra en mi palma abierta y hago una pausa. "Me gusta", murmuro en voz baja. "Me gusta."*

*Mi palma permanece abierta mientras me muevo hacia mi círculo de amigos.*

Author: Noelany Pelc.

## Processing questions for the clients (Preguntas de proceso para los/as clientes)

1. Beyond the overt questions that Paola asked herself, what do you think she was really wrestling with? (*Más allá de las preguntas abiertas que Paola se hizo a sí misma, ¿con qué crees que estaba luchando realmente?*)

2. What would the main character have revealed, when sharing her stone? Take some time to reflect on an item that holds a similar meaning for you. What would others bear witness to, by knowing more about this item? (*¿Qué habría revelado el personaje principal al compartir su piedra? Tómate un tiempo para reflexionar sobre un elemento que tenga un significado similar para ti. ¿De qué darían testimonio los demás al saber más sobre este tema?*)

3. How does the main character balance pride in her stone and what it means to her, and humility and self-compassion in the vulnerability of sharing it with others? (*¿Cómo equilibra el personaje principal el orgullo por su piedra y lo que significa para ella, y la humildad y la autocompasión en la vulnerabilidad de compartirla con los demás?*)

4. What sense do you have, of the conclusion that the main character reached, at the end? In what ways can you see yourself reflected in the conclusion that she reaches? (*¿Qué sentido tiene la conclusión a la que llegó el protagonista, al final? ¿De qué manera te ves reflejada en la conclusión a la que llega ella?*)

## Sayings (*dichos*)

### Saying #1

"Humility is the reflection of the grandeur of your heart and the wealth of your emotions."
*"La humildad es el reflejo de la grandeza de tu corazón y la riqueza de tus sentimientos."*

Author: Unknown. Popular Spanish proverb (J. Vega, personal communication, December 6, 2020).

### Processing questions for the clients (Preguntas de proceso para los/as clientes)

1. Do you perceive your emotions to be a liability or a source of wealth? Elaborate. (*¿Percibe tus emociones como una carga o una fuente de riqueza? Elaborar.*)

2. As a popular proverb, why do you think that this sentiment has resonated with so many? What is the lesson that has been passed down? (*Como dice el proverbio popular, ¿por qué crees que este sentimiento ha resonado con tantos? ¿Cuál es la lección que se ha transmitido?*)

3. What emotion are you most rich in? Why do you think that this proverb ties emotions to humility? (*¿En qué emoción eres más rico? ¿Por qué crees que este proverbio vincula las emociones con la humildad?*)

4. Using the following link, identify three ways in which emotions are adaptive for you. (*Usando el siguiente enlace, identifica tres formas en las que las emociones se adaptan a ti.*)

Link in English: https://nobaproject.com/modules/functions-of-emotions
Link in Spanish: www.divulgaciondinamica.es/blog/emociones-concepto-funciones/

### Saying #2

"Vanity blossoms but bears no fruit."
*"La vanidad florece pero no da fruto."*

Author: Nepalese Proverb (Freeman, 2014).

**Processing questions for the clients (Preguntas de proceso para los/as clientes)**

1. What does this quote mean for you? (*¿Qué significa esta cita para ti?*)
2. In what ways have you pursued praise, perception, validation, or otherwise temporary and fleeting results? Consider, in particular, the efforts you put forth for the benefit of others (e.g., appearances, mannerisms, interests, and so on). What purpose do these efforts serve (e.g., admiration, approval, acceptance)? (*¿De qué manera has perseguido elogios, percepción, validación u otros resultados temporales y fugaces? Considera, en particular, los esfuerzos que realizas en beneficio de los demás (por ejemplo, apariencias, gestos, intereses, etc.). ¿Para qué sirven estos esfuerzos? (por ejemplo, admiración, aprobación, aceptación)*)
3. What dimensions of self do you wish to grow that may produce no visible markers for praise or recognition? Examine. (*¿Qué dimensiones del yo deseas crecer que pueden no producir marcas visibles de elogio o reconocimiento? Examinar.*)

## Quotes

*Quote #1*

"In the course of my life, I have often had to eat my words, and I must confess that I have always found it a wholesome diet."
   *"En el transcurso de mi vida, a menudo he tenido que*
   *Cómete mis palabras, y debo confesar que siempre me ha parecido una dieta sana.".*

Author: Winston Churchill was a British statesman and former Prime Minister (Baron Normanbrook, 1969).

**Processing questions for the clients (Preguntas de proceso para los/as clientes)**

1. Talk about a time when you have had to eat your words. When is it easy to do so, and when is it challenging? (*Habla de un momento en el que hayas tenido que comerte tus palabras. ¿Cuándo es fácil hacerlo y cuándo es un desafío?*)
2. What is your initial response, when you perceive that you have fallen short or made a mistake? How do you communicate these experiences with others? (*¿Cuál es tu respuesta inicial, cuando percibes que te has quedado corto o cometido un error? ¿Cómo comunicas estas experiencias con los demás?*)
3. Picture the last time that you talked about a perceived failure or a mistake. How did you feel, at that moment? Recall the bodily sensations you experienced then, or now (heart rate, posture, where your eye gaze travels, breathing), emotions (fear, shame, peace, etc.), and thoughts. If you are identifying uncomfortable or negative sensations, where do you think that they are coming from? Where did you learn these responses? (*Imagínate la última vez que hablaste sobre un error o un fracaso percibido. ¿Cómo te sentiste en ese momento? Recuerda las sensaciones corporales que experimentaste entonces o ahora (frecuencia cardíaca, postura, hacia donde viaja la mirada, respiración), emociones (miedo, vergüenza, paz, etc.) y pensamientos. Si estás identificando sensaciones incómodas o negativas, ¿de dónde cree que provienen? ¿Dónde aprendiste estas respuestas?*)

4. Identify someone whose responses to errors or mistakes you admire. What do they do well? If you were to create a "formula," based on the positive response(s) that you have witnessed, what would it be? Outline your steps. (*Identifica a alguien cuyas respuestas a los errores o equivocaciones admiras. ¿Qué hacen bien? Si tuviera que crear una "fórmula", basada en las respuestas positivas que ha presenciado, ¿cuál sería? Describe tus pasos.*)

5. When do you not give yourself enough credit? This may require asking others, if you find yourself stuck. (*¿Cuándo no te das suficiente crédito a ti mismo? Esto puede requerir preguntarle a otros, si te encuentras atascado.*)

### Quote #2

"It's like a mother, when the baby is crying, she picks up the baby and she holds the baby tenderly in her arms. Your pain, your anxiety is your baby. You have to take care of it. You have to go back to yourself, to recognize the suffering in you, embrace the suffering, and you get relief."

   "*Es como una madre, cuando el bebé llora, lo levanta y lo sostiene con ternura en sus brazos. Tu dolor, tu ansiedad es tu bebé. Tienes que cuidarlo. Tienes que volver a ti mismo, reconocer el sufrimiento en ti, abrazar el sufrimiento, y obtienes Alivio.*"

Author: Thich Nhat Hanh is a Vietnamese Thien Buddhist Monk, poet, and peace activist (Winfrey, 2017).

### Processing questions for the clients (Preguntas de proceso para los/as clientes)

1. What pain do you carry with you, that is often unrecognized but suffering? (*¿Qué dolor llevas contigo, que a menudo no se reconoce pero sufre?*)

2. If you could give your vulnerability a voice, what would it say to you? Write a letter, from the perspective of your most vulnerable voice. Allow your writing to be unfiltered and unjudged. Write for 10–15 minutes. (*Si pudieras darle voz a tu vulnerabilidad, ¿qué te diría? Escribe una carta, desde la perspectiva de tu voz más vulnerable. Permita que su escritura no esté filtrada ni juzgada. Escribe de 10 a 15 minutos.*)

3. What does this vulnerable voice need? Identify three to four themes, needs, or asks. (*¿Qué necesita esta voz vulnerable? Identifique tres a cuatro temas, necesidades o preguntas.*)

4. What usually prevents you from meeting these needs for yourself? What messages do you hold on to, that prevent you from attending to these needs tenderly? (*¿Qué le impide normalmente satisfacer estas necesidades por sí mismo? ¿A qué mensajes te aferras que te impiden atender con ternura estas necesidades?*)

5. Listen to the "Self-Compassion/Loving-Kindness Meditation" by Dr. Kristen Neff, and identify which parts of the medication come easily to you, and which ones will require more practice. (*Escuche la "Meditación de auto compasión/bondad amorosa" de la Dra. Kristen Neff e identifique qué partes de la medicación le resultan fáciles y cuáles requerirán más práctica.*)

Link in English: https://self-compassion.org/wp-content/uploads/2020/08/LKM.self-compassion_cleaned_01-cleanedbydan.mp3

Link in Spanish: https://bilingualmindfulness.com/es/meditaciones-guiadas/

·)) ⌂  ***Quote #3***

"Because true belonging only happens when we present our authentic, imperfect selves to the world, our sense of belonging can never be greater than our level of self-acceptance."

*"Debido a que la verdadera pertenencia solo ocurre cuando presentamos nuestro yo auténtico e imperfecto al mundo, nuestro sentido de pertenencia nunca puede ser mayor que nuestro nivel de autoaceptación."*

Author: Brené Brown is a U.S.-based researcher, author, professor, and lecturer focusing on themes of self-compassion (2017).

·)) ⌂  **Processing questions for the clients (Preguntas de proceso para los/as clientes)**

1. Find a quiet place where you can be alone. Set aside 20–30 minutes for this exercise. Describe your imperfect self. Write, draw, paint, or otherwise take note of the contradictions that exist within you, the parts of you that you keep to yourself, the parts of you that you struggle with, and so on. This is an exercise for you; even then, it can be difficult to be honest with ourselves. (*Encuentre un lugar tranquilo donde pueda estar solo. Reserva de 20 a 30 minutos para este ejercicio. Describe tu yo imperfecto. Escribe, dibuja, pinta o toma nota de las contradicciones que existen dentro de ti, las partes de ti que te guardas para ti, las partes de ti con las que luchas, etc. Este es un ejercicio para ti; incluso entonces, puede resultar difícil ser honesto con nosotros mismos.*)

2. Take the stance of a benevolent observer. Without judgement or evaluation, observe your reactions to seeing this imperfect self, captured and fully elaborated. What might it be like to love and accept this part of you? Discuss. (*Adopte la postura de un observador benevolente. Sin juzgar ni evaluar, observe sus reacciones al ver este yo imperfecto, capturado y completamente elaborado. ¿Cómo sería amar y aceptar esta parte de ti? Discutir.*)

3. To whom or with whom, do you share this imperfect self? From whom do you obscure these parts of you? In other words, how do you hide yourself from others? Expand. (*¿Con quién o con quién compartes este yo imperfecto? ¿De quién ocultas estas partes de ti? En otras palabras, ¿cómo te escondes de los demás? Expandir.*)

4. What might it be like if someone could peel back the layers that you use for protection, to allow others to see you, as you are? (*¿Cómo sería si alguien pudiera quitar las capas que usas para protegerte, para permitir que otros te vean como eres?*)

## References

Baron Normanbrook, N. C. B. (1969). *Action this day: Working with Churchill.* St. Martin's Press.

Brown, B. (2017, September 11). *Finding our way to true belonging.* TED. https://ideas.ted.com/finding-our-way-to-true-belonging/

Freeman, I. A. (2014). *Seeds of revolution: A collection of axioms, passages and proverbs, volume 1.* iUniverse.

Neff, K. D. (2021). *Fierce self-compassion: How women can harness kindness to speak up, claim their power, and thrive.* Harper Wave.

Winfrey, O. (2017). *The wisdom of Sundays: Life-changing insights from super soul conversations.* Flatiron Books.

# 6 Identity and Intersectionality

Identity can be broadly understood as an expression of self or as a collective social identity. Personal identity can be held internally and is often expressed through comportment, presentation, speech, and a variety of ways in which individuals enact or perform any dimension of themselves. An example of this can be represented by how an individual might perform their gender identity, such that they feel comfortable expressing themselves in ways that feel congruent for them. Collective social identity creates a larger social affiliation with a group, whether that be one's religious (or non-religious), ethnic, racial, gender, country, or larger collective body. For example, individuals may hold strongly to their ethnic identity, but feel distant from their national identity.

Identity, however, is not a singular dimension, and the multiple identities that individuals hold are not separate from one another. Intersectionality refers to the unique lived experiences of individuals, as they move through the world with the overlapping identities that they hold (Crenshaw, 1989). In other words, a Burmese woman who is of high SES, and who has little accent when speaking English will have a different experience in the world than a Burmese woman who is a low SES and has a marked accent when speaking in English. By using an intersectionality framework, mental health providers can more deeply explore how their clients move through the world, how they see themselves, and what systems act upon them, and gather a more complete picture of their client's lived experience. Providers can also explore systems of power and marginalization that may be meaningful in their lives, simultaneously.

*Liberation theory*, or similar consciousness-raising movements, involve the refocusing and centering of voices, identities, histories, and parts of self that are often marginalized in dominant narratives. Often individuals find themselves underrepresented in images, stories, educational materials, and historical information lost or influenced by colonizing or dominant groups. Examining identity often involves the work of re-claiming parts of self that have been lost, marginalized, or uncovered.

See also: relationships, self-realization, self-realization, and courage

 ## Microfiction

### If Flowers Could Sing

". . . A ribbon lies between us, unfurled; bridging the space we have created, welcoming and preparing to embrace each metaphorical flower, and honoring each as a gift to be wrapped. The

DOI: 10.4324/9781003145943-8

first stem spins wildly to the floor—a delicate *anemone* blown in the wind by anticipation and uncertainty. The sociopolitical currents whipping the air around us into a frenzy, carrying sprigs of *cypress* and symbolizing despair—a heavy force crushing the fragile structure of anticipation. Time elapses before a *lavender* stem is solemnly placed on the blanket of despair—silence has crept in. Words elude us. Words perjure us. The royal purple of the *atropa belladona* belies its danger as a *deadly nightshade*. In mere moments, however, a clasped hand thrusts its companion onto the pile, unable to deter the inevitable *bittersweet nightshade* and slamming the silence with its truth—we . . . are . . . still . . . here. An unspoken truth remains a truth. Droplets of water disperse, staining the ribbon in tears shed in private.

Time begins to slow, and for an interminable moment, our eyes meet—but we are not alone. Gentle hands come forth carrying a message of resistance, a *wild tansy* to serve as a beacon. Whispers become hums, and hums become vibrations, and vibrations become songs, carrying voices we had forgotten were present. Lengthy shoots of *statice* are raised, swimming in the crowd and overtaking the space between us. The group raises an ode of remembrance to the women who paved the road before us—a reminder of the history and revolutions that bolster our cause. A rhythm moves into the room, compelling us to capture the movement, swaying and clutching armfuls of *French willow* for bravery and humanity, conducting waves of baskets brimming with *live oak* for liberty, and a powerful surge carrying *edelweiss* reaches the heart of the multitude where the arrangement began—a promise of change and transformation. In the final moments, a shower of *forget-me-nots* flutters to the center, sealing a faithful pact in the face of adversity. Then we work . . .

In unison, we labor over the collective undertaking to swathe each petal, herb, sprig, and stem—insisting on the representative value of each symbolic element, and being equally mindful of the task that unifies us . . ."

(Español)

 **Microficción**

### *Si las Flores Pudieran Cantar*

*"Hay una cinta entre nosotros, desplegada; uniendo el espacio que hemos creado, dando la bienvenida y preparándonos para abrazar cada florete metafórico, y honrando a cada uno como un regalo para envolver. El primer tallo gira violentamente hacia el suelo, un delicado anenomo arrastrado por el viento por la anticipación y la incertidumbre. Las corrientes sociopolíticas azotan el aire a nuestro alrededor en un frenesí, llevando ramitas de ciprés y simbolizando la desesperación, una fuerza pesada que aplasta la frágil estructura de la anticipación. Transcurre el tiempo antes de que un tallo de lavanda se coloque solemnemente sobre el manto de la desesperación; el silencio se ha deslizado. Las palabras nos engañan. La púrpura real de la atropa belladona oculta su peligro como una solanácea mortal. En unos momentos, sin embargo, una mano entrelazada empuja a su compañero sobre la pila, incapaz de disuadir a la inevitable solanácea agridulce y golpeando el silencio con su verdad: nosotros . . . estamos . . . todavía . . . aquí. Una verdad tácita sigue siendo una verdad. Gotas de agua se dispersan, manchando la cinta con lágrimas derramadas en privado.*

*El tiempo comienza a ralentizarse y, por un momento interminable, nuestras miradas se encuentran, pero no estamos solos. Aparecen unas manos suaves que llevan un mensaje de resistencia, un tanaceto salvaje que sirve de faro. Los susurros se convierten en tarareos y los tarareos en vibraciones y las vibraciones en canciones, llevando voces que habíamos olvidado que estaban presentes. Se levantan largos brotes de estática, nadando entre la multitud y superando el espacio entre nosotros. El grupo lanza una oda de recuerdo a las mujeres que allanaron el camino ante nosotros, un recordatorio de la historia y las revoluciones que refuerzan nuestra causa. Un ritmo se mueve en la habitación, obligándonos a capturar el movimiento, balanceando y agarrando brazos de sauce francés por valentía y humanidad, conduciendo oleadas de cestas rebosantes de roble vivo por la libertad, y una poderosa oleada que lleva edelweiss llega al corazón de la multitud donde comenzó el arreglo, una promesa de cambio y transformación. En los momentos finales, una lluvia de nomeolvides revolotea hacia el centro, sellando un pacto de fidelidad ante la adversidad. Entonces trabajamos . . .*

*Trabajamos al unísono en el compromiso colectivo de enhebrar cada pétalo, hierba, ramita y tallo, insistiendo en el valor representativo de cada elemento simbólico y siendo igualmente conscientes de la tarea que nos unifica."*

Author: Noelany Pelc (2017, p. 2).

### Processing questions for the clients (Preguntas de proceso para los/as clientes)

1. Identify the different phases of this short story. What are the themes and catalysts for change? What change occurs from the beginning to the end? (*Identifica las diferentes fases de este cuento. ¿Cuáles son los temas y catalizadores del cambio? ¿Qué cambio ocurre desde el principio hasta el final?*)

2. Take a moment and think about the themes in your life. Make a list of words, feelings, and experiences that capture your own experience of being in the world today. Using this, or a similar tool, www.almanac.com/flower-meanings-language-flowers, browse the meanings of flowers. Create your own metaphorical bouquet that represents your lived experience. Find resources and websites that are relevant for you. This includes searching for culturally specific, historically meaningful, or representative meanings of flowers, herbs, and greenery.

   (*Tómate un momento y piensa en los temas de tu vida. Haz una lista de palabras, sentimientos y experiencias que capturen tu propia experiencia de estar en el mundo de hoy. Usando esta, o una herramienta similar,www.almanac.com/flower-meanings-language-flowers,explora los significados de las flores. Crea tu propio ramo metafórico que represente tu experiencia vivida. Localiza recursos y sitios web que sean relevantes para ti. Esto incluye la búsqueda de significados culturalmente específicos, históricamente significativos o representativos de flores, hierbas y vegetación.*)

3. If a close friend, who loved and knew you, could craft a personalized bouquet for you, what would they thoughtfully include in this gift to you? (*Si un amigo cercano, que te quisiera y te conociera, pudiera elaborar un ramo personalizado para ti. ¿Qué incluirían cuidadosamente en este regalo para ti?*)

4. What elements in your own bouquet, whether your own or that which could be gifted to you, symbolize your own strengths for healing, hope, change, and work? (*¿Qué elementos de tu propio ramo, ya sea el tuyo propio o el que podría regalarse, simbolizan tus propias fortalezas para la curación, la esperanza, el cambio y el trabajo?*)

## Sayings (*dichos*)

### *Saying #1*

"Until the lions have their own historians, the history of the hunt will always glorify the hunter."

"*Hasta que los leones tengan sus propios historiadores, la historia de la caza siempre glorificará al cazador.*"

Author: Chinua Achebe was a Nigerian novelist, poet, and author of *Things Fall Apart* (Brooks, 1994).

### Processing questions for the clients (Preguntas de proceso para los/as clientes)

1. For you, what is the central theme of this saying? (*Para ti, ¿cuál es el tema central de este dicho?*)

*Table 6.1* Representation of Identities in Diverse Forms of Media

| Media (Medios de comunicación) | How were my identities portrayed? (¿Cómo se representaron mis identidades?) | How did I feel about the portrayals I saw/heard/read? (¿Cómo me sentí acerca de las representaciones que vi/escuché/leí?) | What elements of me and my identity(ies) were not shown? (¿Qué elementos míos y de mi (s) identidad (s) no se mostraron?) |
|---|---|---|---|
| Television (Televisión) | | | |
| Films (Películas) | | | |
| Popular literature (fiction and non-fiction) [Literatura popular (ficción y no ficción)] | | | |
| Textbooks or educational materials (Libros de texto o materiales educativos) | | | |
| Music (Música) | | | |

2. Make a list of media that you watched, read, heard, or accessed during your childhood/adolescence. How did this media portray (or not) individuals who share your identities? (*Haz una lista de los medios que viste, leíste, escuchaste o accediste durante tu niñez/adolescencia. ¿Cómo representan (o no) estos medios a las personas que comparten tus identidades?*)

3. Who were you shown to be? What did you learn about yourself through the media? (*¿Quién te demostró ser? ¿Qué aprendiste sobre ti a través de los medios?*)

4. Take 5–10 minutes to reflect on the columns and messages that you received about your identity(ies). What narratives were missing in the media to which you were exposed? (*Tómate entre 5 y 10 minutos para reflexionar sobre las columnas y los mensajes que recibiste sobre tu (s) identidad (es). ¿Qué narrativas faltaban en los medios a los que estuviste expuesto?*)

    a. Identify one or two identities that are most salient for you (e.g., gender, ethnicity, language of origin, ancestral roots, sexual orientation), and read, listen to, or watch a work of art that is authored by someone who shares those identities and speaks to an in-group experience.

    (*Identifica una (1) o dos (2) identidades que sean más destacadas para ti (por ejemplo, género, etnia, idioma de origen, raíces ancestrales, orientación sexual) y lee, escucha o ve una obra por alguien que comparte esas identidades y habla de esta experiencia de grupo.*)

    b. Identify one or two identities that are meaningful for you. Find two or three books, songs, poems, films, or media material that offer a historical perspective or that are informative of sociocultural messages and movements.

    (*Identifica uno o dos identidades que sean significativas para ti. Busca de dos a tres libros, canciones, poemas, películas o material multimedia que ofrezca una perspectiva histórica o que sean informativos de los mensajes y movimientos socioculturales.*)

5. Where do you best find your experience, identity(ies) and voice represented? (*¿Dónde encuentras mejor tu experiencias, identidad (es) y voz representada?*)

 *Cultural Hints*

Within liberation theory, a central goal is to shift the understanding of distress from an intrapersonal and individual concern, to encompass and highlight sociocultural factors that have contributed to and maintained distress (e.g., White supremacy, xenophobia, cis-sexism, transphobia). The use of essays, books, documentaries, and other historically informative materials can offer insight into economic, legislative, political, and historical events that have shaped and contributed to the oppression and marginalization of identities in the United States.

The following electronic resources offer starting points for therapists, counselors, educators, allies, and participants, alike:

1. Equity and Liberation Resources: equity and liberation resources for Black, Indigenous, People of Color, and White allies—www.youthcollaboratory.org/equity-and-liberation-resources

2. Resources for Black Liberation: www.queer-art.org/resources-black-liberation

3. Anti-racism resource collection: www.resourcesharingproject.org/anti-racism-resource-collection

4. Anti-oppression: Anti-transmisia—https://simmons.libguides.com/anti-oppression/anti-transmisia
5. Resources for talking about race, racism, and racialized violence with kids:https://center-racialjustice.org/resources/resources-for-talking-about-race-racism-and-racialized-violence-with-kids/
6. Indigenous Peoples resources: https://indigenouspeoplesresources.com/
7. Resources for Indigenous Peoples: www.culturalsurvival.org/resources

## *Saying #2*

"They tried to bury us. They didn't know we were seeds."
  "*Intentaron enterrarnos. No sabían que éramos semillas.*"

Author: Greek Saying (Syrimis, 1997).

## Processing questions for the clients (Preguntas de proceso para los/as clientes)

1. Identify three moments in time when you felt as though your context or environment attempted to bury you. Take into consideration that this process could be through erasure, systemic oppression, fiscal inequity, among many others. (*Identifica tres momentos en el tiempo en los que sentiste como si tu contexto o ambiente intentara enterrarte. Ten en cuenta que este proceso podría ser a través del borrado, la opresión sistémica, la inequidad fiscal, entre muchos otros.*)
2. Describe what "burying" means to you? How do you feel about these moments? Elaborate on thoughts, feelings, and physiological reactions when you are feeling "buried." (*Describe lo que significa "enterrar" para ti. ¿Cómo te sientes con esos momentos? Explica los pensamientos, sentimientos y reacciones fisiológicas cuando te sientes "enterrado."*)
3. How have you been able to survive and thrive as a seed? What parts of your identity(ies) bolster you and serve as fertilizer for you to flourish? (*¿Cómo has podido sobrevivir y prosperar como semilla? ¿Qué partes de tu (s) identidad (es) te fortalecen y te sirven como fertilizante para que prosperes?*)
4. What are two ways that you can celebrate and honor a part of your identity today? (*¿Cuáles son dos formas en las que puedes celebrar y honrar una parte de tu identidad hoy?*)

## Quotes

## *Quote #1*

1a. "I have come to believe over and over again that what is most important to me must be spoken, made verbal and shared, even at the risk of having it bruised or misunderstood."

  "*He llegado a creer una y otra vez que lo que es más importante para mí debe ser hablado, verbalizado y compartido, incluso a riesgo de que lo lastime o lo malinterprete.*"

1b. "My silences had not protected me. Your silence will not protect you."

  "*Mis silencios no me habían protegido. Tu silencio no te protegerá.*"

Author: Audre Lorde was a self-described "black, lesbian, mother, warrior, poet," who worked as a feminist/womanist civil rights activist and author (Lorde, 2020).

·)) 🎧 **Processing questions for the clients (Preguntas de proceso para los/as clientes)**

1. Read both quotes. Using a writing utensil, circle any words that stand out to you. Underline any words that bring about a strong emotional reaction. Write any of your initial reactions in the margins. What do your markings tell you about what the quotes mean to you? (*Lee ambas citas. Con un utensilio de escritura, encierra en un círculo las palabras que le llamen la atención. Subraya las palabras que provoquen una fuerte reacción emocional. Escribe cualquiera de tus reacciones iniciales en los márgenes. ¿Qué te dicen tus marcas sobre lo que estas citas significan para ti?*)

2. Read the first quote—can you identify parts of yourself that you hold closely, but similarly hide from others? (*Lee la primera cita: ¿puedes identificar partes de ti mismo que tienes de cerca, pero que de manera similar se esconden de los demás?*)

   a. If your silence can take on different forms, how does it manifest in your life? How do you live your life silently? For what purpose? (*Si tu silencio puede tomar diferentes formas, ¿cómo se manifiesta en tu vida? ¿Cómo vives tu vida en silencio? ¿Con qué propósito?*)

   b. What stories about yourself have you not told? What important untold theme would you uncover? (*¿Qué historias sobre ti no has contado? ¿Qué tema importante no contado descubrirías?*)

3. How could you make these stories and themes a central part of your current story? What if you did? Expand. (*¿Cómo podrías hacer de estas historias y temas una parte central de tu historia actual? ¿Y si lo hicieras? Expandir.*)

·)) 🎧 *Quote #2*

"Living on borders and in margins, keeping intact one's shifting and multiple identity and integrity, is like trying to swim in a new element, an 'alien' element."

*"Vivir en las fronteras y en los márgenes, manteniendo intacta la identidad y la integridad cambiantes y múltiples de uno, es como intentar nadar en un nuevo elemento, un elemento 'extraño.'"*

Author: Gloria E. Anzaldua Borderlands/La Frontera: The New Mestiza was a feminist scholar examining Chicana cultural theory and queer theory (2020).

·)) 🎧 **Processing questions for the clients (Preguntas de proceso para los/as clientes)**

1. What do you think Anzaldua meant, when she described the experience of attempting to swim in an "alien" element? (*¿Qué crees que quiso decir Anzaldua cuando describió la experiencia de intentar nadar en un elemento "extraterrestre"?*)

2. Describe your borders and margins—at what points in your story have you felt on the margins? (*Describe tus fronteras y márgenes: ¿en qué puntos de tu historia te has sentido marginado/a?*)

3. Create a map, using any tools, utensils, or mediums that are available to you. Delineate the boundaries, rules, messages, and roles that have shaped the borders. Use color, texture,

words, or any other tools that illustrate your experience. Discuss. (*Crea un mapa, utilizando cualquier herramienta, utensilio o medio que esté disponible para ti. Delinear los límites, reglas, mensajes y roles que han dado forma a las fronteras. Utiliza colores, texturas, palabras o cualquier otra herramienta que ilustre tu experiencia. Discutir.*)

4. If your story had a narrator, how would they narrate the ways in which you have maintained your integrity? What backstory and insights would they offer that aren't always available to you, as the main character? (*Si tu historia tuviera un narrador, ¿cómo se narraría las formas en las que has mantenido tu integridad? ¿Qué historia de fondo e información ofrecerían que no siempre estén disponibles para ti, como personaje principal?*)

### Quote #3

"If I wait for someone else to validate my existence, it will mean that I'm shortchanging myself."

("*Si espero a que alguien más valide mi existencia, significaría que me estoy engañando a mí mismo.*")

Author: Zanele Muholi is a South African activist and artist (2021).

### Processing questions for the clients (Preguntas de proceso para los/as clientes)

1. Who have you been waiting on to validate your existence? Identify how this answer may have changed over your lifespan. (*¿A quién has estado esperando para validar tu existencia? Identifica cómo esta respuesta puede haber cambiado a lo largo de su vida.*)

2. Who or what systems have you allowed to determine your value, experience(s), parts of self, authenticity, and congruence? What have been the benefits and costs? (*¿A quién o qué sistemas has permitido que determine tu valor, experiencia (s), partes de sí mismo, autenticidad y congruencia? ¿Cuáles han sido los beneficios y los costos?*)

3. **Miracle question:** If you woke up tomorrow, and found that you feel fully and authentically yourself—all hesitations and self-judgement are absent—how would you feel differently? Identify how your internal dialogue would change, how your behavior, outlook, goals, and affect would be different. Which message(s) about you would be re-written, if this miracle occurred?

    (***Pregunta milagrosa:*** *Si te despertaras mañana y descubrieras que te sientes plena y auténticamente tu mismo/a y todas las vacilaciones y el juicio propio están ausentes. ¿Cómo te sentirías diferente? Identifica cómo cambiaría tu diálogo interno, cómo sería diferente tu comportamiento, perspectiva, metas y afecto. ¿Qué mensaje (s) sobre ti se volvería a escribir si ocurriera este milagro?*)

## References

Anzaldúa, G. (2012). *Borderlands: The new mestiza= la frontera.* Aunt Lute Books.

Brooks, J. (1994). Chinua Achebe, The art of fiction. *The Paris Review, 139*(133).

Crenshaw, K. (1989). Demarginalizing the intersection of race and sex: A Black feminist critique of antidiscrimination doctrine, feminist theory and antiracist policies. *University of Chicago Legal Forum, 1989*(1), 139–167.

Lorde, A. (2020). *Sister outsider*. Penguin Books.

Muholi, Z. (2021, October 28). www.wisefamousquotes.com/zanele-muholi-quotes/if-i-wait-for-someone-else-to-validate-276255/

Pelc, N. (2017, May). If flowers could sing. *WomenView: The newsletter for the advancement of women in division 17, American Psychological Association*, 2–3. www.div17.org/assets/docs/Womanview-2017-Spring.pdf

Syrimis, G. (1997). [Review of the book Poems]. *Journal of Modern Greek Studies*, *15*(1), 152–154. http://doi.org/10.1353/mgs.1997.0013

# Part II

# **Adversity**

Change and Coping

# 7 Change

Change is at the core of the therapeutic process. When clients are seen, the main expectation is that there will be some type of change at the cognitive, emotional, or behavioral level. Although in principle, change sounds like a simple process, the reality is that for a myriad of reasons human beings are typically resistant to change. Having the ability to change is a sign of conducting self-analysis that results in the implementation of a thought process. Moreover, change is a sign of adaptation to internal and external conditions. Thus, change is normally associated with flexibility and adaptability. When there is a fear of failure, concerns about the future, and expectations, the attitude against change is manifested in the forms of stubbornness, anger, discomfort, avoidance, and defiance. It is the element of resistance to change that few people admit, but which is the basis of this fear. When clients believe that they lack the skills, abilities, or strengths needed to cope with transformation, they often do not admit it, but they react by blocking or sabotaging the transformation process. Helping and guiding a client through the path of change is a slow and complex process that may require lots of patience and support in such a way that the outcome can be seen as a better state than the current situation.

See also: coping, distress tolerance, courage, and patience

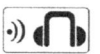 ## Microfiction

### *The Evolution*

In the middle of vast amounts of vegetation, there were a couple of inconspicuous tiny eggs attached to the back of a leaf. The two tiny egg siblings had long conversations amongst themselves. They would talk about the rain that fell on them, the cold drops formed on the leaves in the morning, the sounds of animals, and the power of the sunlight at noon. They experienced many fears as they encountered other insects and birds who were in pursuit of easy prey. They always wondered why they had been left alone glued on a leaf without the protection of their parents. In spite of the fact that they felt defenseless, there was a sense of coziness and protection in their current state as eggs. After all, they did not have to do anything but simply stay on the leaf and wait for things to happen to them. One night, they felt a strange sensation, they were moving inside of the egg and the thin layer started to get brittle until it ruptured. They were outside staring at the world! One of the siblings told the other: "Look at you, you have a long body with tiny legs, am I just like you? The other one replied: "Yes, you are!" Suddenly,

DOI: 10.4324/9781003145943-10

they had a strong urge to move and to eat the flesh of the leaves that they were attached to. They were famished and did not stop eating until the night. Abruptly, a paralyzing fear captured them. "Now we are more vulnerable than ever, birds and big insects can easily spot us as we have bright colors and move slowly," one of the siblings said. The other one said: "Well, let's be smart and use our colors as camouflage as we have the stealthy advantage!" The other sibling refused to move from the spot that he was originally at. As a result, he was running out of leaves to eat and did not have spaces to hide. In the meanwhile, the fearful sibling lost sight of the other. He did not want to move; he wished he was back in the state of an egg in which nothing had to be done but simply be. Facing the fear of movement, he was snatched by a hungry woodpecker. The other sibling kept moving, eating, hiding, and growing. At night, he crawled and cried thinking about the well-being of his sibling. One night he felt an irresistible urge to look for a leaf to rest. He felt as if his body was turning into something solid. Another change! Abruptly, he became petrified, he was not mobile any more. Once again, just like when he was an egg, he was defenseless and at the mercy of the weather, insects, and birds. The only difference was that unlike when he was an egg, now he remembered what it was like to move, be in control, eat, and do the things that he wanted. Once more, he was seeing the world through a thin layer of skin, where everything was blurred. Exactly after 14 days, he started moving inside of this thin pouch, stretching, regenerating, and regaining strength. After a last effort, he saw himself flapping a beautiful pair of colorful wings! Now, he understood everything. A 3,000-mile trip south awaited him. Like having an internal map, some sort of a flying compass, he knew that his destiny was in another place and many adventures awaited him.

(*Español*)

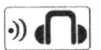 **Microficción**

### *La Evolucion*

*En medio de una gran cantidad de vegetación había un par de discretos y diminutos huevos adheridos al dorso de una hoja. Los dos diminutos huevos hermanos tuvieron largas conversaciones entre ellos. Hablarían de la lluvia que les caería encima, las gotas frías que se formaban en las hojas por la mañana, los sonidos de los animales y el poder de la luz del sol al mediodía. Experimentaron muchos miedos al encontrarse con otros insectos y pájaros que buscaban presas fáciles. Siempre se preguntan por qué los dejaron solos pegados a una hoja sin la protección de sus padres. A pesar del hecho de que se sentían indefensos, había una sensación de comodidad y protección en su estado actual como huevos. Después de todo, no tenían que hacer nada más que quedarse en la hoja y esperar a que les pasaran cosas. Una noche, sintieron una sensación extraña, sus cuerpecillos se estaban moviendo involuntariamente dentro del huevo y la fina capa comenzó a volverse quebradiza hasta que se rompió. ¡Estaban afuera mirando al mundo! Uno de los hermanos le dijo al otro: "Mírate, tienes un cuerpo largo con piernas diminutas, ¿soy como tú? El otro respondió: ¡sí, lo eres! "De repente, sintieron un fuerte impulso de moverse y comer la pulpa de las hojas a las que estaban adheridos. Estaban hambrientos y no dejaron de comer hasta la noche. De repente, un miedo paralizante los capturó. "Ahora somos más vulnerables que nunca, las aves y los insectos grandes pueden vernos fácilmente ya que tenemos colores brillantes y nos movemos lentamente", dijo uno de los hermanos. El otro dijo: "Bueno, ¡seamos inteligentes y usemos nuestros colores como camuflaje ya que tenemos la ventaja de sigilo!" El otro hermano se negó a moverse del lugar en el que estaba originalmente. Como resultado, se estaba quedando sin hojas para comer y no tenía espacios para esconderse. Mientras tanto, el hermano paralizado perdió de vista al otro. No quería moverse, deseaba estar de vuelta en el estado de un huevo en el que no había que hacer nada más que simplemente "ser." Frente al miedo al movimiento, fue secuestrado por un pájaro carpintero hambriento. El otro hermano siguió moviéndose, comiendo, agarrándose y creciendo. Por la noche, se arrastraba y lloraba pensando en el bienestar de su hermano. Una noche sintió un impulso irresistible de buscar una hoja para descansar. Sintió como si su cuerpo se estuviera convirtiendo en algo sólido. ¡Otro cambio! De repente, se quedó petrificado, ya no se movía. Una vez más, al igual que cuando era un huevo, estaba indefenso y a merced del clima, los insectos y los pájaros. La única diferencia era que, a diferencia de cuando era un huevo, ahora recordaba cómo era el moverse, tener el control, comer y hacer las cosas que quería. Una vez más, estaba viendo el mundo a través de una fina capa de piel, todo estaba borroso. Exactamente después de 14 días, comenzó a moverse dentro de esta bolsa delgada, estirándose, regenerándose y recuperando fuerzas. ¡Después de un último esfuerzo, se vio a sí mismo batiendo un hermoso par de alas de colores! Ahora, entendió todo. Un viaje de 3,000 millas al sur lo esperaba. Como teniendo un mapa interno, una especie de brújula voladora, sabía que su destino estaba en otro lugar y le esperaban muchas aventuras.*

Author: Roberto Swazo.

*Cultural Hints*

The concept of change is seen through different cultural filters. For instance, Eastern cultures may see change as going against the cultural traditions that have dominated their collective landscape and therefore, as threatening the status quo. Also, change is put in operation as a group rather than as individuals. As counselors, we must gauge the level of understanding of this concept by the client in such a way that we can evaluate the degree of comfort to exercise change in their lives without putting in danger the principles of their cultures.

**Processing questions for the clients (Preguntas de proceso para los/as clientes)**

1. Which of the two brothers do you identify with? Explain. (*¿Con cuál de los dos hermanos te identificas? Explicar.*)
2. Can you attempt to explain why one of the brothers felt compelled to stay in the same place while the other had the urge to keep going? Discuss. (*¿Puedes intentar explicar por qué uno de los hermanos se sintió obligado a permanecer en el mismo lugar mientras que el otro tenía la urgencia de seguir adelante? Discutir.*)
3. Draw a picture representing both brothers at any stage. Using arrows connecting to their pictures, label the feelings that each brother was feeling. Which feelings are stronger according to you? Elaborate. (*Haz un dibujo que represente a ambos hermanos en cualquier etapa. Usando flechas conectadas a sus dibujos, etiquete los sentimientos que cada hermano estaba sintiendo. ¿Qué sentimientos son más fuertes según tú? Elaborar.*)

## Sayings (*dichos*)

### *Saying #1*

"Better pain for change than stagnation without pain."
*"Más vale dolor por cambio qué estancamiento sin dolor."*

Author: Unknown. Popular Arab saying (K. Ebeid, personal communication, May 21, 2018).

### Processing questions for the clients (Preguntas de proceso para los/as clientes)

1. What is the main point of this quote? Explain. (*¿Cuál es el punto principal de esta cita? Explicar.*)

2. What sort of pains have you experienced in the past that caused you to change? Did the change take you into a positive or negative position in life at that moment? List them and explain. (*¿Qué tipo de dolores has experimentado en el pasado que te hicieron cambiar? ¿El cambio te llevó a una posición positiva o negativa en la vida en ese momento? Enumera y explica.*)

3. Make a list of the times in your life that you have been comfortable with a situation but limited you to progress, grow, or reach the experiences that you always wanted. What would you do differently to prevent stagnation today and why? Explain. (*Haz una lista de los momentos en tu vida en los que te has sentido cómodo con una situación pero te has limitado a progresar, crecer o alcanzar las experiencias que siempre quisiste. ¿Qué harías de manera diferente para evitar el estancamiento hoy y por qué? Explicar.*)

### *Saying #2*

"If the river water changes all the time without protesting, why is it so difficult for us to change ourselves?"
*"Si el agua del río cambia todo el tiempo sin protestar, ¿por qué se nos hace tan difícil cambiarnos a nosotros mismos?"*

Author: Unknown. Popular Jewish saying (S. Rosenbaum, personal communication, June 1, 2018).

### Processing questions for the clients (Preguntas de proceso para los/as clientes)

1. If readily available to you, visit a nearby creek or small river in which the waters are constantly flowing. Take the time to observe the water and all of the dynamics surrounding it. Look at the rocks that have been shaped by the water, debris, leaves, and pieces of branch floating adrift. Pay attention to the obstacles that want to stop the water from flowing and analyze the way the water keeps going organically. What does it say about the way you are handling your own natural path in life? What is blocking you from changing? Describe. (NOTE: if there is no natural creek close to you, access a video link of a creek from YouTube and conduct the exercise.) [*Si está disponible para ti, visita un*

*arroyo cercano o un río pequeño en el que las aguas fluyan constantemente. Tómate el tiempo para observar el agua y toda la dinámica que la rodea. Mira las rocas que han sido moldeadas por el agua, escombros, hojas y trozos de ramas flotando a la deriva. Presta atención a los obstáculos que quieren evitar que el agua fluya y analiza la forma en que el agua sigue fluyendo orgánicamente. ¿Qué dices sobre la forma en que estás manejando tu propio camino natural en la vida? ¿Qué te impide cambiar? Describir. (NOTA: si no hay un arroyo natural cerca de usted, simplemente descárguelo del canal de Youtube y realice el ejercicio).]*

2. Bodies of water are pushed by "invisible" forces that guide them in a graceful way. It is clear that you are destined to move and evolve such as the water does. There is something in you that is serving as an internal compass for change, however, there might be elements that are impeding you to change. Close your eyes and imagine that you are a powerful or a soothing body of water. Nothing can stop it. First, mentally list the things that you want to change and make a note of each one of the items indicating what has stopped you from achieving these. Is this resistance to change coming from what sources? People, events, institutions, or yourself? Read these out loud in front of a mirror. Describe the experience. (*Los cuerpos de agua son empujados por fuerzas "invisibles" que los guían con gracia. Está claro que estás destinado a moverte y evolucionar como lo hace el agua. Hay algo en ti que está sirviendo como una brújula interna para el cambio, sin embargo, puede haber elementos que te impiden cambiar. Cierra los ojos e imagina que eres un cuerpo de agua poderoso o relajante. Nada puede detenerte. Primero, enumera mentalmente las cosas que quieres cambiar y toma nota de cada uno de los elementos indicando qué te ha impedido lograrlos. ¿Esta resistencia al cambio proviene de qué fuentes? ¿Personas, eventos, instituciones o tú mismo? Léelos en voz alta frente a un espejo. Describe la experiencia.*)

## Quotes

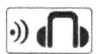

### *Quote #1*

"Everyone thinks of changing the world, but no one thinks of changing himself."
*"Todo el mundo piensa en cambiar el mundo, pero nadie piensa en cambiarse a sí mismo."*

Author: Leo Tolstoy. He was a Russian writer who is regarded as one of the greatest authors of all time. He received nominations for the Nobel Prize in Literature multiple times but never received it (2021).

### Processing questions for the clients (Preguntas de proceso para los/as clientes)

1. Interpret this quote. Can you think of examples of people in your life who have tried to change everyone around them but are unable to do so because they have failed to change themselves? What did you learn from them, be it positive or negative? Elaborate. (*Interprete esta cita. ¿Puedes pensar en ejemplos de personas en tu vida que hayan intentado cambiar a todos los que les rodean, pero no pueden hacerlo porque no han logrado cambiarse a sí mismos? ¿Qué aprendiste de ellos, ya sea positivo o negativo? Elaborar.*)

2. Why is it that you have pointed out the deficiencies in others when you know very well that you need to do it yourself first? Provide examples during different times of your life with different people. (*¿Por qué has señalado las deficiencias en otros cuando sabes muy bien que debes hacerlo tú mismo primero? Proporciona ejemplos durante diferentes momentos de tu vida con diferentes personas.*)

3. If you want to change something in your life or about yourself, the greatest chance of success is based on internal/intrinsic motivation as opposed to external/extrinsic motivation. Now, create a specific plan of action in the form of a table that involves the following: (*Si deseas cambiar algo en tu vida o en ti mismo/a, la mayor posibilidad de éxito se basa en la motivación interna/intrínseca en contraposición a la motivación externa/extrínseca. Ahora, crea un plan de acciones específico en formato de tabla que involucra lo siguiente:*)

*Table 7.1* Reasons for Seeking Change, Plan for Change, and Change in Outlook

| What do I want to change? (*¿Qué quiero cambiar?*) | Why? Is it based on an intrinsic or extrinsic motivation? (*¿Por qué? ¿Se basa en una motivación intrínseca o extrínseca?*) | When do I want to start implementing this? (*¿Cuándo quiero comenzar a implementar esto?*) | When do I want to see the outcome of these changes? (*¿Cuándo quiero ver el resultado de estos cambios?*) | How has the life outlook changed as a result of these changes? (*¿Cómo ha cambiado la perspectiva de la vida como resultado de estos cambios?*) | Additional notes or comments: (*Notas o comentarios adicionales:*) |
|---|---|---|---|---|---|
|  |  |  |  |  |  |
|  |  |  |  |  |  |
|  |  |  |  |  |  |
|  |  |  |  |  |  |

### Quote #2

"The measure of intelligence is the ability to change."
*"La medida de la inteligencia es la capacidad de cambiar."*

Author: Albert Einstein was a Jewish German theoretical physicist who developed the theory of relativity, one of the two pillars of modern physics. His work is also known for its influence on the philosophical aspects of the sciences including ethics (2021).

**Processing questions for the clients (Preguntas de proceso para los/as clientes)**

1. Based on what you know colloquially about Einstein, what message is he trying to convey? Explain. (*Basado en lo que sabes coloquialmente sobre Einstein, ¿qué mensaje está tratando de transmitir? Explicar.*)

2. Sometimes when we do not understand or know something, and therefore we lack information, we experience fear of failure. Failing seems to be part of learning, especially if corrections are made to avoid the same mistakes. What are you afraid of that might involve fear of failure? This could be in the areas of relationships (i.e., romantic, filial, paternal, maternal, social), occupational, relocating, learning a new set of skills, etc. (*A veces, cuando no entendemos o no sabemos algo, y por lo tanto carecemos de información, experimentamos miedo al fracaso. Fallar parece ser parte del aprendizaje, especialmente si se hacen correcciones para evitar los mismos errores. ¿A qué le temes que pueda implicar miedo al fracaso? Esto podría ser en las áreas de relaciones (es decir, romántico, filial, paterno, materno, social), ocupacional, reubicación, aprendizaje de un nuevo conjunto de habilidades, etc.*)

3. We are hardwired to resist change at all costs. The amygdala in our brain tends to decode change as a threatening force resulting in the release of the hormones for fear, fight, or flight. Therefore, the structures in your body want to protect you from change. Exercise: Go back to the table created in Exercise #3 of Quote #1 and select the first item from the list. Mentally, picture yourself going through the process of change. Imagine that you are executing this with full details. Describe the body sensations connected to this particular change event. Start with how your breathing changes, sudoration, palpitations, GIS (gastrointestinal symptoms), mental images, etc. Try to reset yourself mentally with a successful mental picture. Start with minor changes and increase these gradually as you get more comfortable. (*Estamos programados para resistir el cambio a toda costa. La amígdala en nuestro cerebro tiende a decodificar el cambio como una fuerza amenazante que resulta en la liberación de hormonas para el miedo, la lucha o la huida. Por lo tanto, las estructuras de tu cuerpo quieren protegerte del cambio.*

   *Ejercicio: Regresa a la tabla creada en el Ejercicio n. ° 3 de la Cita n. ° 1 y selecciona el primer elemento de la lista. Mentalmente, imagínate atravesando el proceso de cambio. Imagina que estás ejecutando esto con todos los detalles. Describe las sensaciones corporales conectadas a este evento de cambio en particular. Comienza con el cómo cambia tu respiración, sudoración, palpitaciones, SIG (síntomas gastrointestinales), imágenes mentales, etc. Intenta restablecerte mentalmente con una imagen mental exitosa. Comienza con cambios menores y aumenta estos gradualmente a medida que te sientas más cómodo/a.*)

*Quote #3*

"Change is the law of life, and those who look only to the past and present are certain to miss the future."

"*El cambio es la ley de la vida, y aquellos que solo miran al pasado y al presente seguramente se perderán el futuro.*"

Author: John Fitzgerald Kennedy was an American politician who served as the 35th president of the United States from January 1961 until his assassination in November 1963 (1963).

### Processing questions for the clients (Preguntas de proceso para los/as clientes)

1. How are the past, present, and future intertwined when it comes to change in our lives? Analyze. (*¿Cómo se entrelazan el pasado, el presente y el futuro cuando se trata de cambios en nuestras vidas? Analizar.*)
2. According to this quote, "change is the law of life," how would you interpret this? (*Según esta cita, "el cambio es la ley de la vida", ¿cómo interpretarías esto?*)
3. In nature, change is an organic process that takes place at all times. There is a change of seasons, plants and animals go through distinctive phases of development, the planet changes, and the universe expands. Overall, change is a constant and not a variable. There are four barriers to change in human beings: work environments, old (unhelpful) habits, attachments to mindsets and worldviews, and the attitude toward learning. Which of these appear to be the greatest barrier for change in your life? Of these, what can be changed the fastest? Elaborate. (*En la naturaleza, el cambio es un proceso orgánico que tiene lugar en todo momento. Hay un cambio de estaciones, las plantas y los animales pasan por distintas fases de desarrollo, el planeta cambia y el universo se expande. En general, el cambio es una constante y no una variable. Hay cuatro barreras para el cambio en los seres humanos: entornos de trabajo, viejos (malos) hábitos, apegos a las mentalidades y visiones del mundo, y la actitud hacia el aprendizaje. ¿Cuál de estos parece ser el mayor obstáculo para el cambio en tu vida? De estos, ¿cuál se puede cambiar más rápido? Elaborar.*)

### References

Einstein, A. (2021, May 17). https://readingjunction.com/measure-intelligence-ability-change/

Kennedy, J. F. (1963, June 25). *Address in the Assembly Hall at the Paulskirche in Frankfurt (266). Public papers of the presidents: John F. Kennedy, 1963.* The American Presidency Project. www.presidency.ucsb.edu/documents/address-the-assembly-hall-the-paulskirche-frankfurt

Tolstoy, L. (2021, May 17). *Full text of Pamphlets. Translated from the Russian 1900.* https://archive.org/stream/pamphletstransl00tolsgoog/pamphletstransl00tolsgoog_djvu.tXt

# 8  Adversity

Adversity is seen as an event or combination of situations that has brought difficulty or suffering to an individual or group of people. Normally, it is associated with a catastrophic event, but also exists in day-to-day challenges. Since human beings perceive reality in a subjective way, occasionally, individuals describe one event as a catastrophe while others see it as a minor "bump on the road." Perhaps the best way to describe adversity is to contextualize it according to a common reality that creates some type of objective parameter. For example, if a multimillionaire loses 1 million dollars during the collapse of the stock market, it will simply be a beep on the radar. On the other hand, for common folks who have worked all their lives and were able to save 1 million dollars through their 401(K), losing 1 million dollars would mean losing everything that they have worked for and therefore, depleting their retirement funds completely. Similarly, a farmer who has 30 cows that fell ill to a lethal virus and consequently died, it would mean that his family will lose their source of income. A megafarm can lose hundreds of cattle and will quickly recuperate due to their diverse portfolio of investments. Then, adversity is contextual to the reality of different individuals. For some, adversity can be a gift and an opportunity to explore new horizons, while for others it can be a cause for immobilization. For some, it is an opportunity to build character and develop while for others it is a catalyst to developing resentment and impacting relationships with those around them. The greatest challenge for human services providers is to acknowledge the pain of a unique perception, while empowering the individual to move forward and use this event as a catalyst for change and personal development.

See also: criticism, coping, courage, distress tolerance, and future

 ## Microfiction

### *Stronger Than Bullets*

Hunger, pain, discrimination, oppression, and despair were the daily doses of my existence. The mere act of peeking through the window was an exercise of bravery. It seems like the first 15 years of my life were a distant past, a blurred memory that was a false illusion rather than the recollection of true events. I remember going to school with my friends, laughing, enjoying life, and embracing life at its fullest. All the kids and families in the neighborhood attended family gatherings, birthday parties, and religious events regardless of personal affiliations. Life was

DOI: 10.4324/9781003145943-11

good, no financial scarcity, all basic needs were met, and the outlook of the future was good. However, things started to slowly change as the result of the breakup of the Socialist Federal Republic of Yugoslavia. Suddenly, resentments among ethnic and religious groups resurfaced from nowhere. Abruptly, Bosnian Muslims and Catholic Croats were seen as inferior and the enemy to the Orthodox Serbian national and ethnic identity. As a young adolescent, I was not involved in politics or religion, and it was hard for me to comprehend why many of my friends stopped talking to me. Schools started to close, basic goods were scarce, people were beaten up on the streets, and graffiti was sprayed on the doors of the apartments of Bosnian and Croat families. Papa was shot dead on the street by a sniper on his way back from his construction work.

I saw him lying down on the ground like a mannequin from the window of our apartment for three days before a couple of family members were able to retrieve his body. My oldest brother died as a result of a brutal beating perpetrated by a mob of nationalists. It was just mama and I, both imprisoned in our apartment like vulgar criminals. They had cut the gas and electricity; therefore, we could not heat up whatever scraps we had for food. Snipers terrorized us day and night. People were shot like wild ducks as if our lives were worth nothing. Some neighbors were shot through the windows! So, mama did not let me peek through the window during the day. Only at night, when no one can see our silhouettes, did I have the valor to peek through the window to see what was left of my previous world. Mama started to get weaker and weaker and she ran out of her medications for her respiratory condition. We had no food. We were cold and slowly dying of hunger. I had no option but to venture outside and try to get to some food at our relatives' apartments. I know that some of our uncles and aunts had taken off to Germany as refugees while others left for America. Papa always believed that everything was going to eventually get better. It never did.

One night, I ventured outside in order to look for some bread at one of our friend's apartments. I remember being so weak that I had to take breathing breaks every 25 meters. My clothes were hanging as I was merely a collection of bones and skin. No, no, no! When I came back, mama was on the floor in a fetal position with a face full of peace. Her skin was as pale as a ghost. No breathing, movement. Mama was gone! My relatives were gone, friends had managed to move out of the area, and our apartment building smelled like death. I decided to stay put for a few days. Mama's body started to smell, the entire apartment smells like rotten meat. I started to sleep most of the day, I had no energy, and no strength left to cry. Everything was a blur. I had to look for help outside. I managed to go downstairs and started crawling around the garbage and objects in the yard. Suddenly, the light became darkness, pain turned into numbness. I could not feel my legs and one arm was paralyzed. I lay down for a full day and thought about mama's smell in the apartment and papa's body on the ground for days.

Ten days after, I do not remember how I got here, and who helped me but I am at a refugee camp in Germany with the intent to be shipped to America. I have been told that I will not be able to walk and have permanently lost one arm. After all, who needs legs when I can run as far as I want with my imagination? Who needs an additional arm when I can type, write, and draw with one? The sky is blue; everything smells fresh; and I have food, people around me who care about my life, and a future to help others avoid the pitfalls of hate. After all, I can change more people with my story and experiences than the average person. I have the power to change an entire generation. There is no room for rage, revenge, or war but for transformation. What else can I ask for?!

(*Español*)

## Microficción

### *Más Fuerte Que Las Balas*

*El hambre, el dolor, la discriminación, la opresión y la desesperación fueron las dosis diarias de mi existencia. El mero acto de mirar por la ventana fue un ejercicio de valentía. Parece que los primeros 15 años de mi vida fueron un pasado lejano, un recuerdo borroso que fue una falsa ilusión más que el recuerdo de hechos reales. Recuerdo ir a la escuela con mis amigos, reír, disfrutar de la vida y abrazar la vida al máximo. Todos los niños y las familias del vecindario asistían a reuniones familiares, fiestas de cumpleaños y eventos religiosos, independientemente de sus afiliaciones personales. La vida era buena, no había escasez financiera, se satisfacían todas las necesidades básicas y las perspectivas para el futuro eran buenas. Sin embargo, las cosas empezaron a cambiar lentamente como resultado de la desintegración de la República Federativa Socialista de Yugoslavia. De repente, los resentimientos entre grupos étnicos y religiosos surgieron de la nada. De repente, los musulmanes bosnios y los croatas católicos fueron vistos como inferiores y enemigos de la identidad étnica y nacional serbia ortodoxa. Cuando era adolescente, no estaba involucrado en política ni religión, y era difícil para mí comprender por qué muchos de mis amigos dejaron de hablarme. Las escuelas empezaron a cerrar, los productos básicos escaseaban, la gente fue golpeada en las calles y se rociaron grafitis en las puertas de los apartamentos de familias bosnias y croatas. Papá fue asesinado a tiros en la calle por un francotirador cuando regresaba de su trabajo de construcción. Lo vi tirado en el suelo como un maniquí desde la ventana de nuestro apartamento durante tres días antes de que un par de miembros de la familia pudieran recuperar el cuerpo. Mi hermano mayor murió como resultado de una brutal golpiza perpetrada por una turba de nacionalistas. Solo éramos mamá y yo, ambos encarcelados en nuestro apartamento como delincuentes vulgares. Habían cortado el gas y la electricidad, por lo tanto, no pudimos calentar las sobras de comida que teníamos. Los francotiradores nos aterrorizaban día y noche. A la gente le disparaban como patos salvajes tal y como si nuestras vidas no valieran nada. ¡Algunos vecinos recibieron disparos por las ventanas! Por lo tanto, mamá no me dejó mirar por la ventana durante el día. Solo por la noche, cuando nadie podía ver nuestras siluetas, tuve el valor de asomarme por la ventana para ver lo que quedaba de mi mundo anterior. Mamá comenzó a debilitarse cada vez más y se le acabaron los medicamentos para su afección respiratoria. No teníamos comida. Teníamos frío y moríamos lentamente de hambre. No tuve más remedio que aventurarme a salir e intentar conseguir algo de comida en los apartamentos de nuestros familiares. Sé que algunos de nuestros tíos y tías se habían marchado a Alemania como refugiados, mientras que otros se habían ido a Estados Unidos. Papá siempre creyó que todo iba a mejorar con el tiempo. Nunca ocurrió así.*

*Una noche, me aventuré a salir a buscar pan en el apartamento de uno de nuestros amigos. Recuerdo que estaba tan débil que tenía que hacer pausas para respirar cada 25 metros. Mi ropa colgaba ya que era simplemente una colección de huesos y piel. ¡No no no! Cuando regresé, mamá estaba en el suelo en posición fetal con el rostro lleno de paz. Su piel estaba tan pálida como un fantasma. Sin respiración, sin movimiento. ¡Mamá se había ido! Mis parientes se habían ido, los amigos habían logrado mudarse del área y nuestro edificio de apartamentos olía a muerte. Decidí quedarme unos días. Mamá empezó a apestar, todo el apartamento huele a carne podrida. Empecé a dormir la mayor parte del día, no tenía energía y no me quedaban fuerzas para llorar. Todo estaba borroso. Tuve que buscar ayuda afuera. Me las arreglé para bajar las escaleras y comencé a arrastrarme alrededor de la basura y los objetos en el patio. De repente, la luz se convirtió en oscuridad, el dolor en entumecimiento. No podía sentir mis piernas y un brazo estaba paralizado. Me acosté durante todo un día y pensé en el olor de mamá en el apartamento y el cuerpo de papá en el suelo durante días.*

*Diez días después, no recuerdo cómo llegué aquí y quién me ayudó, pero estoy en un campo de refugiados en Alemania con la intención de que me envíen a Estados Unidos. Me han dicho que no podré caminar y que he perdido un brazo de forma permanente. Después de todo, ¿quién necesita piernas cuando puedo correr todo lo que quiero con mi imaginación? ¿Quién necesita un brazo adicional cuando puedo mecanografiar, escribir y dibujar con uno? El cielo es azul, todo huele fresco, tengo comida, gente a mi alrededor que se preocupa por mi vida y un futuro para ayudar a otros a evitar las trampas del odio. Después de todo, puedo cambiar a más personas con mi historia y experiencias que la persona promedio. Tengo el poder de cambiar a toda una generación. No hay lugar para la rabia, la venganza o la guerra, sino para la transformación. ¿Qué más puedo pedir?*

Author: Roberto Swazo.

## *Cultural Hints*

For some cultures, adversity can be seen as a predetermined plan for their lives. Or, some may interpret it as the punishment for actions taken by them or ancestors. Moreover, some cultures and religious groups might see adversity as an opportunity to grow in patience and humanity. Hence, adversity may be explicated in terms of a sign from a higher power that current ways of living must be changed. Likewise, instead of trying to alter the conditions of adversity, some will embrace it as an accepted reality. For Western oriented cultures, adversity is interpreted and analyzed as a series of unfortunate events that cannot be changed; however, one's attitude toward them can make a significant difference.

### Processing questions for the clients (Preguntas de proceso para los/as clientes)

1. Put yourself in the shoes of the main character of the story. Can you describe the rainbow of feelings that you would be experiencing if these events were happening to you? Explain. (*Ponte en la piel del personaje principal de la historia, ¿puedes describir el arcoíris de sentimientos que estarías experimentando si estos eventos te estuvieran sucediendo? Explicar.*)

2. Speculate about the evolution of perspectives that the character had (from survival and pessimism to positive transformation) and how in spite of all the tragic events, she became such a powerful human being. (*Especula sobre la evolución de perspectivas que tuvo el personaje (desde la supervivencia y el pesimismo hasta la transformación positiva) y cómo a pesar de todos los trágicos acontecimientos se convirtió en un ser humano tan poderoso.*)

3. On a scale from 1–10 (10 being the highest positive feeling), what are your typical reactions to adverse situations? Are you able to overcome these initial negative reactions on your own or do you need outside sources to help you process the events? (*En una escala del 1 al 10 (siendo 10 el sentimiento positivo más alto), ¿cuáles son tus reacciones típicas ante situaciones adversas? ¿Eres capaz de superar estas reacciones negativas iniciales por tu cuenta o necesitas fuentes externas que te ayuden a procesar los eventos?*)

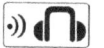 **Sayings (*dichos*)**

 *Saying #1*

"Difficulties make you a jewel."
   "*Las dificultades te convierten en una joya.*"

Author: Unknown. Japanese saying (A. Sato, personal communication, March 12, 2019).

 **Processing questions for the clients (Preguntas de proceso para los/as clientes)**

1. What is the key message of this quote? Explain. (*¿Cuál es el mensaje clave de esta cita? Explicar.*)
2. What is your personal definition of adversity, and how do you typically handle adversity in your life? Elaborate. (*¿Cuál es tu definición personal de adversidad y cómo manejas normalmente la adversidad en tu vida? Elaborar.*)
3. Normally, it takes time, labor, and challenges to bring up the jewel to its splendor. For instance, the melting point of gold is 1,948 degrees Fahrenheit (1,064°C), and the boiling point occurs at 5,173 degrees Fahrenheit. In order to achieve this degree of malleability, one has to have the right equipment and conditions. Diamonds form from pure carbon in the mantle of earth under extreme heat and pressure. Likewise, in order to produce a diamond to be mounted on a ring, the jeweler has to work long hours to refine and polish it. Where are you in the process of evolution (melting gold or pure carbon) towards the perfection of the jewel in you? And, how do you handle the stages of adversity in your life that would produce a jewel in you? Provide details. (*Normalmente, lleva tiempo, trabajo y desafíos hacer que la joya alcance su esplendor. Por ejemplo, el punto de fusión del oro es de 1.948 grados Fahrenheit (1.064 ° C) y el punto de ebullición se produce a 5.173 grados Fahrenheit. Para lograr este grado de maleabilidad, uno tiene que tener el equipo y las condiciones adecuadas. Los diamantes se forman a partir de carbón puro en el manto de la tierra bajo calor y presión extremos. Asimismo, para producir un diamante y para montarlo en un anillo, el joyero tiene que trabajar muchas horas para refinarlo y pulirlo. ¿Dónde estás en el proceso de evolución (fundiendo oro o carbón puro) hacia la perfección de la joya que hay en ti? Y, ¿cómo manejas las etapas de adversidad en tu vida que producirían una joya en ti? Proporcionar detalles.*)

 *Saying #2*

"Smooth seas do not make skillful sailors."
   "*Mares tranquilos no hacen marineros hábiles.*"

Author: Unknown. African saying (Holmes, n.d.).

 **Processing questions for the clients (Preguntas de proceso para los/as clientes)**

1. What is the main teaching point of this quote? Explain. (*¿Cuál es el principal punto de enseñanza de esta cita? Explicar.*)

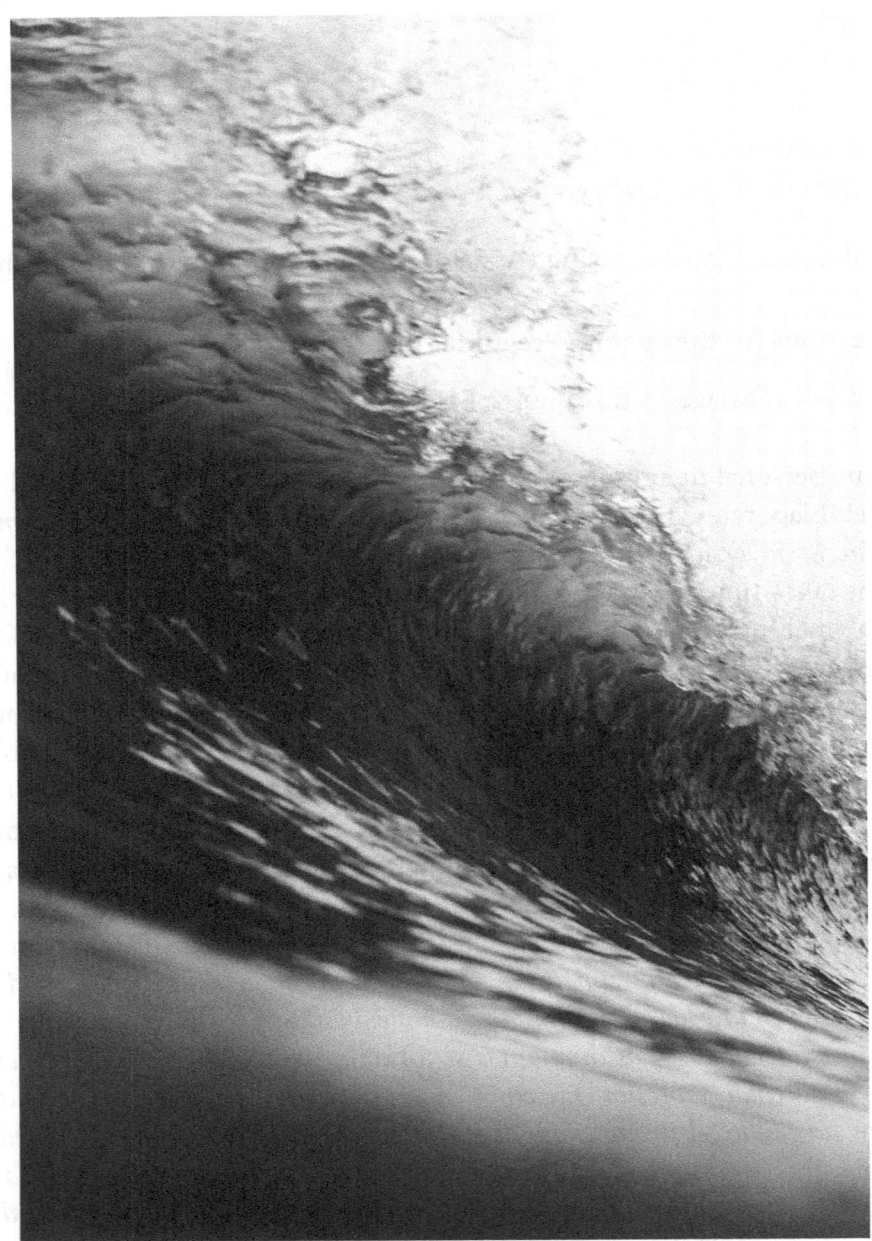

*Figure 8.1* Rough Seas

2.  Analyze the picture that follows. If you were on your own facing the rough waves in an open sea, aside from trying to swim and survive, how would your outlook of life change if you survived it? Describe. (*Analiza la imagen de abajo. Si estuvieras solo frente a las fuertes olas en un mar abierto, además de intentar nadar y sobrevivir, ¿cómo cambiaría tu perspectiva de la vida si lo sobrevivieras? Describir.*)

3.  How are people who suffer from adversity different from those who have had a sheltered life? Explain. (*¿En qué se diferencian las personas que sufren adversidades de las que han tenido una vida protegida? Explicar.*)

## Quotes

### *Quote #1*

"Something very beautiful happens to people when their world has fallen apart: a humility, a nobility, a higher intelligence emerges at just the point when our knees hit the floor."

("*Algo muy hermoso le sucede a la gente cuando su mundo se ha derrumbado: una humildad, una nobleza, una inteligencia superior emerge justo en el momento en que nuestras rodillas golpean el suelo*".)

Author: Marianne Williamson (2013). She is a bestselling author, political activist, and spiritual thought leader.

### Processing questions for the clients (Preguntas de proceso para los/as clientes)

1. Based on your personal experience, what is the relationship between adversity and humility? Elaborate. (*Según tu experiencia personal, ¿cuál es la relación entre la adversidad y la humildad? Elaborar.*)

2. Have you ever experienced an adverse/tragic/difficult event that changed your perspective of life, relationships with others, and the world around you in general? How do you keep this new perspective alive? Explain. (*¿Alguna vez has experimentado un evento adverso/trágico/difícil que cambió tu perspectiva de la vida, las relaciones con los demás y el mundo que lo rodea en general? ¿Cómo mantienes viva esta nueva perspectiva? Explicar.*)

3. From the following options, which ones resemble the most your perspective about adversity in life? You can select more than one. Explain your answers.

    a. Tragedies are a natural consequence of our present circumstances and past actions.
    b. Tragedies are sent by a higher being to test our faith.
    c. Tragedies are sent by a higher power to punish us.
    d. Tragedies are pre-determined by forces out of our control.
    e. Tragedies can serve as a learning tool to grow and develop other areas of our lives.
    f. Only bad people suffer from tragedies in life.

    (*De las siguientes opciones, ¿cuál se parece más a tu perspectiva sobre la adversidad en la vida? Puedes seleccionar más de uno. Explica tus respuestas.*

    a. *Las tragedias son una consecuencia natural de nuestras circunstancias presentes y acciones pasadas.*
    b. *Las tragedias son enviadas por un ser superior para probar nuestra fe.*
    c. *Las tragedias son enviadas por un poder superior para castigarnos.*
    d. *Las tragedias están predeterminadas por fuerzas fuera de nuestro control.*
    e. *Las tragedias pueden servir como una herramienta de aprendizaje para crecer y desarrollar otras áreas de nuestra vida.*
    f. *Solo las personas malas sufren tragedias en la vida.*)

**Quote #2**

"If the only tool you have is a hammer, you tend to see every problem as a nail." ("*Si la única herramienta que tiene es un martillo, tiende a ver cada problema como un clavo.*")

Author: Abraham Maslow (2002).

**Processing questions for the clients (Preguntas de proceso para los/as clientes)**

1. "Attitude is sometimes stronger than circumstances." Based on this quote, create the following plan:

   a. On a daily basis, keep track of your self-talk, even for minor or mundane daily transactions.
   b. Attempt to track the moments in which you use irrational or self-defeating language that serves as an obstacle to overcome difficult moments in life.
   c. Keep a tally of the specific cognitive language and metamessages, stop when they come to your mind, and immediately substitute them with positive ones.
   d. After one week, reevaluate your progress, repeat, and perfect the self-talk techniques in order to overcome these self-defeating thoughts.

   ("*La actitud a veces es más fuerte que las circunstancias.*"
   *Con base en esta cita, crea el siguiente plan:*

   a. *Diariamente, realiza un seguimiento de tu diálogo interno, incluso para transacciones diarias menores o mundanas.*
   b. *Intenta rastrear los momentos en los que utilizas un lenguaje irracional o contraproducente que te sirve de obstáculo para superar los momentos difíciles de la vida.*
   c. *Lleva un registro del lenguaje cognitivo específico y de los metamensajes; detente cuando estos ocurran y sustitúyelos inmediatamente por otros positivos.*
   d. *Después de una semana, reevalúa tu progreso, repite y perfecciona las técnicas de diálogo interno para superar estos pensamientos contraproducentes.*)

2. Conduct a library or web search and look for autobiographies of individuals who overcame adversity, conquered it, and became more actualized human beings. Make a list of the mechanisms and strategies that they used to overcome these. Create your own mechanisms as an adaption of the strategies from these individuals. Keep them in a place that you can read them every morning before you start your day. (*Realiza una búsqueda en la biblioteca o en la web y busca autobiografías de personas que han superado la adversidad, la han conquistado y se han convertido en mejores seres humanos. Haz una lista de los mecanismos y estrategias que utilizaron para superarlos. Crea tus propios mecanismos como una adaptación de las estrategias de estos individuos. Guárdalos en un lugar donde puedas leerlos todas las mañanas antes de comenzar el día.*)

3. Identify three individuals who you admire. Research these individuals, their family origins, surrounding cultures, obstacles, and conditions that were pervasive in their time. Target their "inner minds" and replicate their worldviews and motivations to overcome adversity.

*(Identifica a tres personas a las que admiras. Investigue a estos individuos, sus orígenes familiares, las culturas circundantes, los obstáculos y las condiciones que dominaban en su época. Apunte a sus "mentes internas" y reproduzca sus visiones del mundo y motivaciones para superar la adversidad.)*

### Quote #3

"Out of adversity comes opportunity."
   *"De la adversidad surge la oportunidad."*

Author: Benjamin Franklin (2003).

**Processing questions for the clients (Preguntas de proceso para los/as clientes)**

1. Based on the preceding quote, what is your definition of opportunity in life? Can you provide a series of examples that illustrate this in your life? (*Según la cita anterior, ¿cuál es tu definición de oportunidad en la vida? ¿Puedes proporcionar una serie de ejemplos que ilustran esto en su vida?*)

2. Let's try the **problem-free talk technique in your life**. Imagine that you _____ (fill the blank with a challenging event or adversity such as: have been laid off from work after been in a company for 20 years, got a note of eviction from your rental place, receive a note that your home will be foreclosed in 90 days, your significant other wants to break up with you, your dog of 15 passed away, your son, daughter, mother or father died tragically, etc.). After the normal grieving process, try to speak for a full day as if there were no problems or concerns. Try to reboot your brain and flush it out from negative thoughts or debris. Now, this is the tricky one, based on this tragic event or adversity, how can you take advantage of this to embrace a new and exciting opportunity in your life? Be as specific as possible.

   (*Intentemos la **técnica de hablar sin problemas en tu vida**. Imagine que tu _____ (llene el espacio en blanco con un evento desafiante o adversidad como: has sido despedido del trabajo después de haber estado en una empresa durante 20 años, recibiste una nota de desalojo de tu lugar de alquiler, recibiste una nota de que tu casa será ejecutado en 90 días, tu pareja quiere romper con contigo, tu perro de 15 años falleció, tu hijo, hija, madre o padre murió trágicamente, etc.). Después del proceso normal de duelo, intenta hablar durante un día completo como si no hubiera problemas o preocupaciones. Intenta reiniciar su cerebro y elimínalo de pensamientos negativos o escombros. Ahora, este es el truco, basado en este trágico evento o adversidad, ¿cómo puedes aprovechar esto para aprovechar una nueva y emocionante oportunidad en tu vida? Se lo más específico posible.*)

3. Look at the picture that follows. Make a list of all the adversities that this seed had to go through in order to germinate and be a new plant in the middle of a sea of concrete. If that little seed could overcome so many challenges and obstacles, don't you think that you have all the innate abilities, tools, and courage to imitate this little miracle in the

plant? Be concrete, and list all the strengths that you have and how these can be implemented during moments of adversity in your life. Discuss. (*Mira la foto de abajo. Haz una lista de todas las adversidades que tuvo que atravesar esta semilla para poder germinar y ser una nueva planta en medio de un mar de concreto. Si esa pequeña semilla pudo superar tantos desafíos y obstáculos, ¿no crees que tienes todas las habilidades, herramientas y coraje innatas para imitar este pequeño milagro en la planta? Se concreto y enumera todas las fortalezas que tienes y cómo se pueden implementar durante los momentos de adversidad en tu vida. Discutir.*)

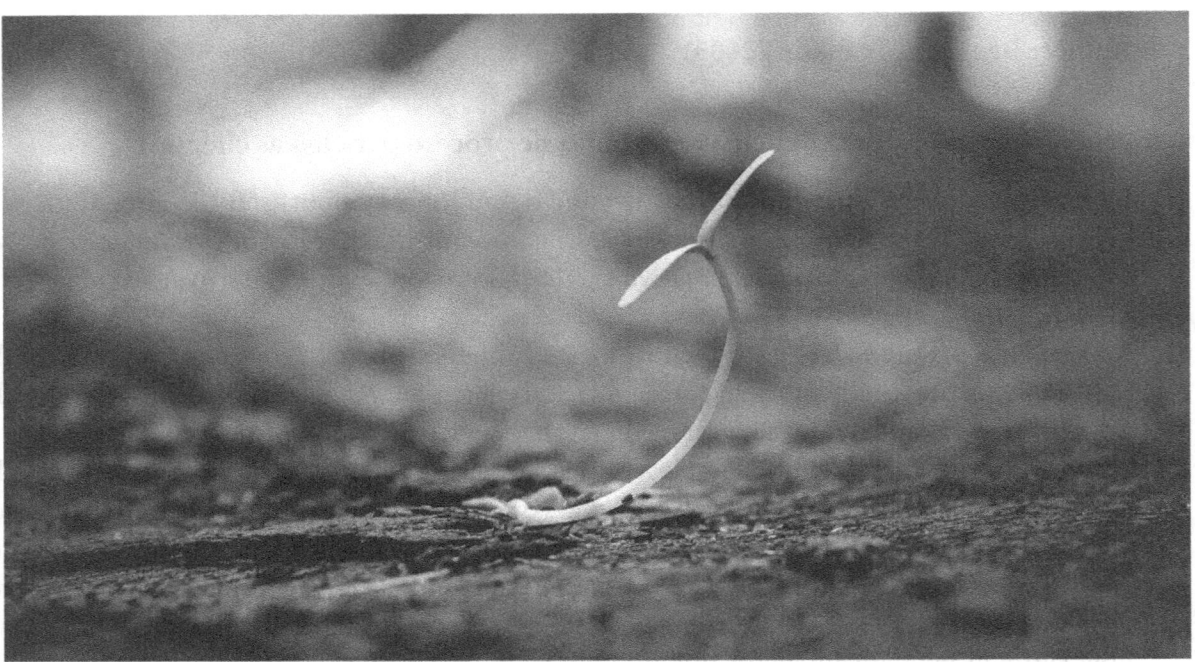

*Figure 8.2* Small Seedling Sprouting in Barren Soil

 *Cultural Hints*

While the concept of adversity is addressed as an existential concern in many of these quotes, it is important to consider real physical, financial, safety, housing, and other basic needs that must be addressed before and/or concurrently. For some individuals, adversity is an ongoing part of their everyday lives. Highlighting resilience that has already been cultivated or is evident in the lives of clients can serve as a reframing for clients who experience shame and hopelessness.

## References

Franklin, B. (2003). *Quotations of Benjamin Franklin*. Applewood Books.

Holmes, D. (n.d.). *African proverbs*. Sayings and Words of Wisdom in English. www.noblepath.info/sayings_and_words_of_wisdom/sayings_and_words_of_wisdom.pdf

Maslow, A. (2002). *The psychology of science: A reconnaissance*. https://b-ok.cc/book/2515438/87bdaa

Williamson, M. (2013, August 31). I've had the great privilege in my life of working with those who suffer [Status update]. *Facebook*. www.facebook.com/williamsonmarianne/posts/10153175865970580

# 9   Health

Health is a multidimensional construct that spans a spectrum of physiological, psychological, spiritual, relational, and developmental dimensions. Our understanding of health, wellness, and quality of life is uniquely influenced by the cultural context and setting in which health is being examined. Culture and sociocultural positionality, such as age, gender, and socioeconomic status often shape the expectations that we hold around pain, quality of life, coping with health changes, treatment recommendations, where individuals seek treatment, and the understanding of the origins of illness.

Similarly, the cultural backdrop informs norms related to care for those who are ill, and appropriate emotional expressions of pain, sadness, grief, fear, anger, and any other myriad of normal reactions to changes in health or ability status. For example, in the United States, it is socially acceptable for men to show anger, but less acceptable to demonstrate fear or hopelessness. Conversely, women are expected to demonstrate fear, tearfulness, and uncertainty, but receive social pressure to avoid expressing anger, which is normative when experiencing grief or loss. Additionally, the internal experience of feeling or being diagnosed as unwell is a uniquely personal journey. Illness or threat of illness often triggers a jarring confrontation with mortality, and a reassessing of our purpose, value, and reflection of our lives. While aging is a natural developmental phase across many cultures, Western culture often ties the movement into older adulthood to loss and deterioration, and medicalizes the care of older individuals.

See also: change, trust, change, future, motivation, and hope

 ## Microfiction

### The Gift of Health

I amble down the sidewalk, yearning to keep pace with the movement around me. My steps falter and I brace myself against the movements of the stream of passersby who seem to be racing. Why so fast? The wind snaps my scarf, lifting the lengthy ends as if urging me to reach my destination. There was a time when not even the wind could make demands of me. Today, every muscle, ligament, tendon, and bone compels me to the wooden bench at the edge of the park. At the edge of everything, really. I stamp my numbing legs involuntarily, as if to punish the sidewalk for the unexpected challenge it presents. I heave a deep and unsteady breath, unwinding the scarf wrapped loosely around my neck and tugging at the fingers of my gloves.

DOI: 10.4324/9781003145943-12

I feel the crisp breeze tickle its way around my exposed neck and fingers, gently announcing that winter is not yet at an end.

My eyes fall to my lap, framing hands that appear curiously translucent under the midday sun. The folded hands open to my gaze, unfurling under my scrutiny, as if allowing themselves to be measured, quantified, and judged. I am lost in a map of textures and roads, paths that wind down leathery hills, only to end abruptly in a crosshatch of creased ravines. There was a time when these paths were silken roads, a decorative pattern of lines engraved rather than etched. There was a time when the ache that is ever present seemed distant, or did it ever exist at all? Was there a time when these fingers worked of their own accord, rather than with my determined persuasion?

All at once, my hands feel timeless in the memories kept between these fingers; the thread they have delicately spun, knots expertly reversed, fingers that have counted, caressed, and patiently woven masterpieces. The masterpieces that lie next to me on the bench; the masterpieces that I chained, stitched, and purled into animation, lifeless now that they have been removed. A moment in time, a different time, a collection of times that span decades of masterpieces.

The playful yipping of a pup engrossed in his defiance of leash training calls me to the present. Instinctively, I draw my gloves close, hiding my fingers from the elements. My fingers shift to find the warmth encased in the gloves, admiring the royal blues and teals swirled together into the stiches. Deliberately, albeit adeptly, working to fasten the decorative bows sustaining the fabric at the top of my wrists. The golden loops dangle and remind me of bows, presents, and special days.

(*Español*)

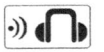 **Microficción**

### El Regalo de la Salud

*Camino por la acera, anhelando seguir el ritmo del movimiento a mi alrededor. Mis pasos vacilan y me preparo contra los movimientos de la corriente de transeúntes que parecen correr. ¿Por qué tan rápido? El viento zarandea mi bufanda, levantando los extremos largos como si me instara a llegar a mi destino. Hubo un tiempo en el que ni siquiera el viento podía controlarme. Hoy, cada músculo, ligamento, tendón y hueso me obligan a subir al banco de madera al borde del parque. Al borde de todo, de verdad. Golpeo involuntariamente mis piernas entumecidas, como para castigar a la acera por el desafío inesperado que presenta. Respiro profundo e inestable, desenrollando la bufanda que me envuelve holgadamente alrededor del cuello y tirando de los dedos de mis guantes. Siento que la brisa fresca se abre paso alrededor de mi cuello y mis dedos expuestos, anunciando gentilmente que el invierno aún no ha terminado.*

*Mis ojos se posan en mi regazo, enmarcando unas manos que parecen curiosamente translúcidas bajo el sol del mediodía. Las manos cruzadas se abren ante mi mirada, desplegándose bajo mi escrutinio, como si se permitieran medir, cuantificar y juzgar. Estoy perdido en un mapa de texturas y caminos, senderos que serpentean por colinas esquivas, solo para terminar abruptamente en un entramado de barrancos arrugados. Hubo un tiempo en que estos caminos eran caminos de seda, un patrón decorativo de líneas grabadas en lugar de grabadas. Hubo un momento en que el dolor que siempre está presente parecía distante, ¿o alguna vez existió? ¿Hubo un momento en que estos dedos trabajaron por sí mismos, en lugar de con mi decidida persuasión?*

*De repente, mis manos se sienten atemporales en los recuerdos guardados entre estos dedos, el hilo que han tejido con delicadeza, los nudos hábilmente invertidos, los dedos que han contado, acariciado y tejido con paciencia obras maestras. Las obras maestras que se encuentran a mi lado en el banco; las obras maestras que encadené, cosí y convertí en animación, sin vida ahora que han sido eliminadas. Un momento en el tiempo, un tiempo diferente, una colección de épocas que abarcan décadas de obras maestras.*

*El ladrido juguetón de un cachorro absorto en su desafío al entrenamiento con correa me llama al presente. Instintivamente, acerco mis guantes, ocultando mis dedos de los elementos. Mis dedos se mueven para encontrar la calidez encerrada en los guantes, admirando los azules reales y los verdes se arremolinan juntos en los puntos de sutura. Deliberadamente, aunque hábilmente, trabajando para sujetar los lazos decorativos que sostienen la tela en la parte superior de mis muñecas. Los lazos dorados cuelgan y me recuerdan a lazos, regalos y días especiales.*

Author: Noelany Pelc.

 **Processing questions for the clients (Preguntas de proceso para los/as clientes)**

1. Identify two or three parts of your body that have served as gifts for you. What have they helped you create, achieve, build, construct, or imagine? (*Identifica dos a tres partes de tu cuerpo que te hayan servido de regalo. ¿Qué te ha ayudado a crear, lograr, construir, construir o imaginar?*)

2. Draw a timeline that is lengthy enough for you to draw and write details into. Mark meaningful events related to health (positive and challenging). No detail is too small or large, if it has been impactful in your health story. (*Dibuja una línea de tiempo que sea lo suficientemente larga para que puedas dibujar y escribir detalles. Marca eventos significativos relacionados con la salud (positivos y desafiantes). Ningún detalle es demasiado pequeño o grande si ha tenido un impacto en tu historia de salud.*)

   Tip: You can also choose to focus on important periods of time related to health. (*Consejo: también puedes optar por centrarte en períodos de tiempo importantes relacionados con la salud.*)

3. What aspects of your health consume you? Create a list of phrases, statements, and thoughts that often pop into your head (e.g., "this isn't fair" or "why me?"). Next to your list, identify the feelings that you associate with each of these thoughts or statements. It is likely that you have multiple feelings attached to each statement. Which ones bubble to the surface? (*¿Qué aspectos de tu salud te consumen? Crea una lista de frases, afirmaciones y pensamientos que a menudo te vienen a la cabeza (por ejemplo, "esto no es justo" o "¿por qué a mí?"). Junto a tu lista, identifica los sentimientos que asocias con cada uno de estos pensamientos o declaraciones. Es probable que tengas varios sentimientos adjuntos a cada declaración. ¿Cuáles salen a la superficie?*)

**Sayings (*dichos*)**

 *Saying #1*

> "Sickness tells us what we are."
> > "*La enfermedad nos dice lo que somos.*"

Author: Unknown. Popular Italian Proverb (2021).

 **Processing questions for the clients (Preguntas de proceso para los/as clientes)**

1. If you were to give your illness or health concerns a voice, what does it tell you about yourself? Describe the voice, tone, pitch, and intent. (*Si tuvieras que dar voz a tu enfermedad o problemas de salud, ¿qué te dice sobre ti? Describe la voz, el tono, el tono y la intención.*)

2. Look inside yourself and find a countervoice. Even a small or quiet one will do. What response(s) does this voice offer? What would it say about you that is similar or different from the voice of your illness? (*Mira dentro de tí mismo y encuentra una contra voz. Incluso una pequeña o silenciosa servirá. ¿Qué respuesta (s) ofrece esta voz? ¿Qué diría de ti que sea similar o diferente a la voz de tu enfermedad?*)

3. You will need a reflective surface, preferably a mirror, and a dry erase marker or other washable marking utensil. Look at yourself in the mirror and reflect on what your health concerns have unearthed or revealed about you. Write them on the margins of your mirror or paper nearby. (*Necesitará una superficie reflectante, preferiblemente un espejo y un marcador de borrado en seco u otro utensilio de marcado lavable. Mírese en el espejo y reflexione sobre lo que sus preocupaciones de salud han descubierto o revelado sobre usted. Escríbalos en los márgenes de su espejo o papel cercano.*)

   a. What are you made of? Focus on internal characteristics. (*¿De qué estás hecho? Céntrate en las características internas.*)

   b. What aspects of you have surprised you, in a positive way? (*¿Qué aspectos de ti te han sorprendido de manera positiva?*)

   c. What has helped you cope as you manage your health? (*¿Qué te ha ayudado a sobrellevar la situación mientras manejas tu salud?*)

   d. How have your priorities changed, if at all? (*¿Cómo han cambiado tus prioridades, si es que han cambiado?*)

4. Think of the last time that you did not feel burdened by your health concerns, even for a moment? What did it feel like? What were you thinking? What was different? Homework: Identify a song that best represents this mood for you. (*¿Piensa en la última vez que no te sentiste agobiado por tus preocupaciones de salud, ni siquiera por un momento? ¿Qué sentiste? ¿Qué estabas pensando? ¿Qué fue diferente? Tarea: Identifica una canción que represente mejor este estado de ánimo para ti.*)

*Saying #2*

"For the unlearned, old age is winter; for the learned, it is the season of the harvest."
*"Para los ignorantes, la vejez es invierno; para los sabios, es la temporada de la siega."*

Author: Unknown. Popular Hasidic Saying (2021).

**Processing questions for the clients (Preguntas de proceso para los/as clientes)**

1.  What seeds did you plant across your life that you are reaping today? Imagine sorting the fruits of your labor into categorical baskets such as: relationships, work, service, spiritual growth, hurdles, ideas, etc. (*¿Qué semillas plantaste a lo largo de tu vida que estás cosechando hoy? Imagínate el clasificar los frutos de tu trabajo en cestas categóricas como: relaciones, trabajo, servicio, crecimiento espiritual, obstáculos, ideas, etc.*)
2.  What fruits of your labor have yet to be harvested? How can you nurture and tend to these crops? (*¿Qué frutos de tu trabajo aún no se han cosechado? ¿Cómo puedes cuidar estos cultivos?*)
3.  When do the days feel like winter for you? What aspects of your health and ability feel most present during these seasons of winter? (*¿Cómo te parecen los días de invierno? ¿Qué aspectos de tu salud y capacidad se sienten más presentes durante estas temporadas de invierno?*)
4.  Make a chart with two columns, one for aspects of your health that *are*, and one for aspects of your health as you *want* them to be. Rank them in order (1–10; with 1 being the least and 10 being the most), according to which prompt the most urgency. (*Haz una tabla con dos columnas, una para los aspectos de tu salud que son reales y otra para los aspectos de su salud como tu quieres que sean. Clasifícalos en orden (del 1 al 10; siendo 1 el menor y 10 el mayor), según el motivo de mayor urgencia.*)

*Saying #3—COVID-19 Specific*

"One moment of patience may ward off a great disaster. One moment of impatience may ruin a whole life."
*"Un momento de paciencia puede evitar un gran desastre. Un momento de impaciencia puede arruinar una vida entera."*

Author: Unknown. Popular Chinese Proverb (2021).

**Processing questions for the clients (Preguntas de proceso para los/as clientes)**

1.  What do you see as your personal responsibility, in keeping your community healthy? (*¿Cuál crees que es tu responsabilidad personal para mantener la salud de tu comunidad?*)
2.  What measures do you take, to ward off great disasters? (*¿Qué medidas tomas para evitar grandes desastres?*)

3.  What is the responsibility of your neighbors and community members, in managing the spread of COVID-19? To what extent do you trust your community to keep you safe? (*¿Cuál es la responsabilidad de tus vecinos y miembros de la comunidad en el manejo de la propagación de COVID-19? ¿Hasta qué punto confías en que tu comunidad te mantendrá a salvo?*)

4.  When is it difficult for you to observe the recommended health and safety guidelines in your area? (*¿Cuándo te resulta difícil observar las pautas de salud y seguridad recomendadas en tu área?*)

    a.  When do you find yourself most impatient to see the pandemic resolve? (*¿Cuándo te sientes más impaciente por ver que la pandemia se resuelva?*)

    b.  How does your impatience influence the decisions that you make? (*¿Cómo influye tu impaciencia en las decisiones que tomas?*)

5.  Do an Internet search using a reputable news source, to identify the number of cases and deaths accurate as of today. Using a sheet of paper, make two columns and label them: "pros" and "cons." Make a thorough list of the pros of following the recommended safety and health guidelines for your area, and cons of violating the guidelines recommended. What personal and community implications arise? (*Realiza una búsqueda en la Internet utilizando una fuente de noticias acreditada para identificar la cantidad de casos y muertes precisas hasta el día de hoy. Con una hoja de papel, haz dos columnas y etiquétalas: "pros" y "contras". Haz una lista completa de las ventajas de seguir las pautas de seguridad y salud recomendadas para tu área y las desventajas de violar las pautas recomendadas. ¿Qué implicaciones personales y comunitarias surgen?*)

 *Cultural Hints*

In some communities of the United States, trust in the medical and scientific community has eroded. Similarly, the individual and collective beliefs about roles and responsibilities during the COVID-19 pandemic can vary dramatically depending on political stance, geographic location, and individualistic/collectivistic worldview. Health carries a spectrum of definitions according to the cultural context of the individual(s). It can be measured across spiritual, emotional, relational, physical, genetic, collective, fiscal, and psychological domains and is best evaluated and assessed in the context of these other variables. Beliefs about health, access to healthcare, and cultural health practices shape how clients will approach health-related goals. Inquiring about health practices, beliefs about origins of health, trusted providers, and familial traditions of wellness and antidotes can build trust and advance therapeutic goals.

## Quotes

 *Quote #1*

"There is no old age. There is, as there always was, just you."
    "*No hay vejez. Estás, como siempre, solo tú.*"

Author: Carol Matthau. She was an American actress and author (1993).

**Processing questions for the clients (Preguntas de proceso para los/as clientes)**

1. What parts of you have remained consistent over the course of your life? If you were introducing a character with these core elements of self to others, how would you describe them? Focus on internal and external traits that have persisted. Examples could be: outlook of the world, personality, temperament, values, hair texture. (*¿Qué partes de ti se han mantenido constantes a lo largo de tu vida? Si estuvieras presentando un personaje con estos elementos centrales de uno mismo a otros, ¿cómo los describirías? Concéntrate en los rasgos internos y externos que han persistido. Los ejemplos podrían ser: perspectiva del mundo, personalidad, temperamento, valores, textura del cabello.*)

2. What has been the theme of your life story? What common threads have persisted in the plot of your life story? Identify the title and design a cover page that best capture your life themes. You can choose to draw, paint, color, or find images on the Internet for your cover page. (*¿Cuál ha sido el tema de tu historia de vida? ¿Qué hilos comunes han persistido en la trama de tu historia de vida? Identifica el título y diseña una portada que capture mejor los temas de tu vida. Puedes elegir dibujar, pintar, colorear o buscar imágenes en la Internet para tu portada.*)

 *Quote #2*

"A Man's illness is his private territory and, no matter how much he loves you and how close you are, you stay an outsider. You are healthy."

"*La enfermedad de un hombre es su territorio privado y, no importa cuánto te ame y cuán cerca estés, te mantienes como un extraño. Estás sano.*"

Author: Lauren Bacall. She was an American actress (1985).

 **Processing questions for the clients (Preguntas de proceso para los/as clientes)**

1. In what ways have you felt isolated from others who cannot share your internal experience of health or aging? Describe. (*¿De qué manera te has sentido aislado de otros que no pueden compartir tu experiencia interna de salud o envejecimiento? Describir.*)

2. Using any medium (e.g., paint, colored pencils, ripped paper, stones, sand, charcoal, graphic design), illustrate your private territory. What parts of your territory remain unexplored? What does your landscape look like and what does each element represent for you? (*Utilizando cualquier medio (por ejemplo, pintura, lápices de colores, papel rasgado, piedras, arena, carbón, diseño gráfico), ilustra tu territorio privado. ¿Qué partes de tu territorio quedan sin explorar? ¿Cómo es tu paisaje y qué representa cada elemento para ti?*)

3. Imagine an oasis hidden in your territory. What parts of your territory serve as your oasis? Where does it reside? What is housed there? How do you nurture the oasis, in moments when it feels like other parts of your territory are overtaking your place of peace and rest? (*Imagina un oasis escondido en tu territorio. ¿Qué partes de tu territorio te sirven de oasis? ¿Dónde residen? ¿Qué se aloja allí? ¿Cómo nutres el oasis en momentos en los que te sientes como si otras partes de tu territorio se apoderaran de tu lugar de paz y descanso?*)

4. If there were a bridge that could help to connect others to you, and vice versa, to your internal territory, what would it be? Bridges could include words spoken, feelings, actions, or other forms of connecting, and can also include a combination of items. (*Si hubiera un puente que pudiera ayudar a conectar a otros contigo, y viceversa, con tu territorio interno, ¿cuál sería? Los puentes pueden incluir palabras habladas, sentimientos, acciones u otras formas de conexión, y también pueden incluir una combinación de elementos.*)

### Quote #3

"Illness is the night side of life, a more onerous citizenship. Everyone who is born holds dual citizenship, in the kingdom of the well and in the kingdom of the sick. Although we all prefer to use a good passport, sooner or later each of us is obliged, at least for a spell, to identify ourselves as citizens of that other place."

"*La enfermedad es el lado nocturno de la vida, una ciudadanía más onerosa. Todo el que nace tiene doble ciudadanía, en el reino de los sanos y en el reino de los enfermos. Aunque todos preferimos usar un buen pasaporte, tarde o temprano cada uno de nosotros está obligado, al menos por un rato, a identificarnos como ciudadanos de ese otro lugar.*"

Author: Susan Sontag, "Illness as Metaphor." She is an American philosopher, activist, and author (2013).

1. In your travels with the more "onerous citizenship," what elements of your health do you find yourself avoiding? Which are easiest for you to manage? What do you think prompts the differences in responses. Identify one or two items that are important to your well-being, and accessible to you, but that elicit strong emotional responses (e.g., avoidance, anger, frustration, exhaustion). [*En tus viajes con la "ciudadanía más onerosa", ¿qué elementos de tu salud evitas? ¿Cuáles te resultan más fáciles de gestionar? ¿Qué crees que provoca las diferencias en las respuestas? Identifica de uno a dos elementos que son importantes para tu bienestar y accesibles para ti, pero que provocan fuertes respuestas emocionales (por ejemplo, negación, enojo, frustración, agotamiento).*]
2. What do you pack in your suitcase when you travel to the kingdom of the well? (*¿Qué llevas en tu maleta cuando viajas al reino del pozo?*)
3. What items are necessary for you when you travel to the kingdom of the sick? What do you wish you could pack to bring with you? Who do you trust to travel with you? (*¿Qué elementos son necesarios para ti cuando viajas al reino de los enfermos? ¿Qué te gustaría poder llevar contigo? ¿En quién confías para viajar contigo?*)
4. Even when you are in the kingdom of the sick, in what ways do you hold on to your dual citizenship? What aspects of your life remind you that you hold residency in both kingdoms? (*Incluso cuando estás en el reino de los enfermos, ¿de qué manera te aferras a tu doble ciudadanía? ¿Qué aspectos de tu vida te recuerdan que tienes residencia en ambos reinos?*)

## References

Bacall, L. (1985). *Lauren Bacall by myself*. Random House Publishing Group.

Chinese Proverb. (2021, February 4). www.quotespedia.org/authors/c/chinese-proverbs/one-moment-of-patience-may-ward-off-great-disaster-one-moment-of-impatience-may-ruin-a-whole-life-chinese-proverb/

Hasidic Saying. (2021, March 3). www.quoteslyfe.com/quote/For-the-unlearned-old-age-is-winter-260046

Italian Proverb. (2021, April 1). www.bartleby.com/89/1572.html

Matthau, C. (1993). *Among the porcupines: A memoir*. Random House Publishing Group.

Sontag, S. (2013). *Illness as metaphor and AIDS and its metaphors*. Penguin Books Limited.

# 10 Death and Grief

Death has been conceptualized as a distinctive and separate entity from life in Western culture. By and large, death has been depicted as a dark force associated with a Machiavellian dimension that seeks to judge human beings with eternal punishment or rewards depending on one's behavior on earth. Contingent on one's set of beliefs, death can be seen as an extension of life or the culmination of existence and eradication of consciousness. Invariably, death signifies the disconnection with loved ones and the inevitable assessment of one's existence, meaning and purpose of life. As a result, and because of the unknown of the afterlife, death can be a source of existential anxiety and disquietude. Assisting clients with the conceptualization of death is a powerful journey.

See also: change, distress tolerance, coping, and peace

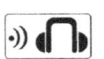 ## Microfiction

### *The Question*

The woman was unable to achieve sleep. Day after day she was consumed with the question of when was going to be the last day for her on this earth. She consulted with her genetic counselor and inquired about her family history pertaining to longevity, congenital diseases, and ways to prolong and defeat any potential illnesses. Finally, she decided to pursue a period of asceticism which entailed a retreat of isolation and meditation that lasted for months. Her goal was to find out when was going to be her last day on earth. The answer had to come from some source, internally or externally. To her surprise, one evening after a long day of prayers and meditations she heard a Voice that whispered to her soul. "Why do you want to know when you will die?" She responded, "Because I really need to know how much time I have left. That is all." The Voice answered, "If I tell you when your last day on earth will be, there are two possible scenarios that you could encounter: (a) nothing and no one, and as a result, will be consumed by the years, months, days, hours, minutes, and seconds left in your life. As a result you will stop working, creating, producing, and doing good things on this earth, or (b) you will follow a path of self-destructive behavior and engage in irresponsible behaviors and do lots of damage to yourself and others. As a result, enjoy your life, be responsible with the gift given to you, and make every minute of your existence count."

(*Español*)

DOI: 10.4324/9781003145943-13

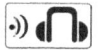 **Microficción**

*La Pregunta*

*La mujer no podía conciliar su sueño. Día tras día estaba consumida por la pregunta de cuándo iba a ser el último día en esta tierra para ella. Ella consultó con su asesor genético y le preguntó sobre sus antecedentes familiares relacionados con la longevidad, las enfermedades congénitas y las formas de prolongar y vencer cualquier enfermedad potencial. Finalmente, decidió seguir un período de ascetismo que implicaba un retiro de aislamiento y meditación que duró meses. Su objetivo era averiguar cuándo iba a ser su último día en la tierra. La respuesta tenía que venir de alguna fuente, interna o externa. Para su sorpresa, una noche después de un largo día de oraciones y meditaciones, escuchó una Voz que le susurró a su alma: "¿Por qué quieres saber cuándo vas a morir?" Ella dijo: "Porque realmente necesito saber cuanto tiempo me queda, eso es todo". La Voz dijo: "Si te digo cuándo será tu último día en la tierra, estos son los dos posibles escenarios que enfrentarás: (a) nada ni nadie, y al pasar de los años, meses, días, horas, minutos y segundos serás consumida por los que quedan en tu vida. Como resultado, dejarás de trabajar, crear, producir y hacer cosas buenas en esta tierra, o (b) seguirás un camino de comportamiento autodestructivo y participarás en comportamientos irresponsables y te harás mucho daño a ti misma y a los demás. Como resultado, disfruta de tu vida, sé responsable con el regalo que recibes y haz que cada minuto de tu existencia cuente."*

Author: Roberto Swazo.

 *Cultural Hints*

In some cultures, religion and spirituality are used as coping mechanisms to conceptualize the duality of life and death. And death to some is seen as a reward to a better level of existence. Similarly, in most Eastern religions, death is not seen as the "end of life" but as an extension of it. Therefore, the clinician must ascertain the client's beliefs and cultural tenets to attempt to comprehend the impact of death in his/her life. Additionally, morning rituals vary from culture to culture, and what can be depicted as unusual or bizarre by Western clinicians falls within the normalcy parameters of other cultures.

 **Processing questions for the clients (Preguntas de proceso para los/as clientes)**

1. What was your initial "gut" reaction after reading this microfiction? (*¿Cuál fue tu reacción inicial "visceral" después de leer esta microficción?*)
2. Why do you think the woman was consumed with the idea of dying? (*¿Por qué crees que la mujer se consumió con la idea de morir?*)
3. How frequently do you think about dying? What are the triggers that make you think about death? Are these fleeting thoughts or do you dwell on them? Do you think that you need psychological help, or is it normal to consider? (*¿Con qué frecuencia piensas en morir? ¿Cuáles son los desencadenantes que te hacen pensar en ello? ¿Son estos pensamientos fugaces o te detienes a pensar en ellos? ¿Crees que necesitas ayuda psicológica o es normal?*)
4. Do you feel that you are in denial of your limited existence on this earth? Explain. (*¿Sientes que estás negando tu existencia limitada en esta tierra? Explica.*)

5. If you knew exactly when you were going to die, regardless if it is far from today or not (i.e., specific year, day, time, location), how would your current daily activities change as a result of this piece of information? What would you do differently with respect to: *(Si supiera exactamente cuándo iba a morir, independientemente de si está lejos de hoy o no (es decir, año, día, hora, ubicación específicos), ¿cómo cambiarían sus actividades diarias actuales como resultado de esta información? ¿Qué haría diferente con respecto a:)*

   a. relationships with loved ones (i.e., friends, family, co-workers, etc.). [*Relaciones con seres queridos (es decir, amigos, familiares, compañeros de trabajo, etc.).*]
   b. daily activities. (*Actividades diarias.*)
   c. work and productivity. (*Trabajo y productividad.*)
   d. leisure. (*Ocio.*)

## Sayings (*dichos*)

### Saying #1

"Everything is missing for those who are alive, and all is left over for those who are dead."
   "*A los vivos todo le falta y a los muertos todo le sobra.*"

Author: Unknown. Popular Latin American saying (J. Delgado, personal communication, February 7, 2017).

### Processing questions for the clients (Preguntas de proceso para los/as clientes)

1. Make a list of everything that is missing in your life. (*Haz una lista de todo lo que falta en tu vida.*)
2. From the previous list, rank the items based on personal versus social value. (*De la lista anterior, clasifique los elementos según el valor personal o social.*)
3. How many of these items are you taking with you after your death? Explain. (*¿Cuántos de estos artículos llevas contigo después de tu muerte? Explique.*)

### Saying #2

"Ultimately, all of us were born to die."
   "*Al fin y al cabo todos nacimos para morir.*"

Author: Unknown. Latin American saying (J. Delgado, personal communication, February 7, 2017).

### Processing questions for the clients (Preguntas de proceso para los/as clientes)

1. If death is the only certainty in life, what is the reason that you were born? (*Si la muerte es la única certeza en la vida, ¿cuál es la razón por la que naciste?*)
2. How do you find meaning on a daily basis? (*¿Cómo encuentras significado diariamente?*)

3. Generate a list of the things that give you purpose to live. How many of these are people, objects, events, or natural cycles? Elaborate. (*Genere una lista de las cosas que le dan un propósito para vivir. ¿Cuántos de estos son personas, objetos, eventos o ciclos naturales? Elabore.*)

## Quotes

 ### Quote #1

"Death is something we should not fear because, while we are, death is not, and when death is, we are not."

"*La muerte es algo que no debemos temer porque, mientras somos, la muerte no es, y cuando la muerte es, nosotros no somos.*"

Author: Antonio Machado, Spanish poet and one of the leading figures of the Spanish literary movement known as the Generation of '98 (2011).

**Processing questions for the clients (Preguntas de proceso para los/as clientes)**

1. How do you interpret the meaning of this quote? (*¿Cómo interpretas el significado de esta cita?*)
2. Are you afraid of dying or living? Explain. (*¿Tienes miedo de morir o vivir? Explica.*)
3. If living is the opposite of dying, what prevents you from enjoying life fully? (*Si vivir es lo opuesto a morir, ¿qué te impide disfrutar plenamente de la vida?*)

### Quote #2

"Death is only important to the extent that it makes us reflect on the value of life."

"*La muerte sólo tiene importancia en la medida que nos hace reflexionar sobre el valor de la vida.*"

Author: André Malraux, French novelist, art theorist, and Minister of Cultural Affairs (Malraux, 2021).

**Processing questions for the clients (Preguntas de proceso para los/as clientes)**

1. How frequently do you reflect on the value of life? Elaborate. (*¿Con qué frecuencia reflexionas sobre el valor de la vida? Elabora.*)
2. If life is the most valuable commodity, make a list of the times, things, and people that you are thankful for living. Elaborate. (*Si la vida es el bien más valioso, haga una lista de las veces, cosas y personas por las cuales está agradecido por vivir. Elaborar.*)
3. How do you celebrate life on a daily basis without infringing upon the rights, values, and boundaries of others? (*¿Cómo celebras la vida a diario sin infringir los derechos, valores y límites de los demás?*)

*Quote #3*

"If death were not the prelude to another life, the present life would be cruel mockery."
*"Si la muerte no fuera el preludio a otra vida, la vida presente sería una burla cruel."*

Author: Mahatma Gandhi, Indian lawyer, politician, social activist, and writer who became the leader of the nationalist movement against the British rule of India (2021).

 *Cultural Hints*

This is a classic example of Eastern philosophies and the principle of reincarnation which radically departs from the theists religions (i.e., Judaism, Christianity, and Islam). The exploration of Eastern beliefs and the interpretation of an ephemeral period of existence viewed as a stage of refinement and development is an important tenet among many religions. As a therapist, one may take advantage of this principle and have a strong reasoning for exploring all possible tools that will make the client live a more fulfilling life.

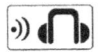 **Processing questions for the clients (Preguntas de proceso para los/as clientes)**

1. What is the main message by the author? (*¿Cuál es el mensaje principal del autor?*)
2. Explain the beliefs that you hold about what occurs after your physical death. (*Explica las creencias que tienes sobre lo que ocurre después de tu muerte física.*)
3. Where are these beliefs coming from? (*¿De dónde vienen estas creencias?*)
4. Were these values imposed by others? Or, have you engaged in a serious process of analysis and reflections that eventually led to an ownership process? (*¿Fueron estos valores impuestos por otros? ¿O has participado en un proceso serio de análisis y reflexiones que eventualmente condujo a un proceso de auto-propiedad?*)

## References

Gandhi, M. (2021, June 18). https://quotestats.com/topic/quotes-about-death-by-gandhi/

Machado, A. (2011). *Times alone: Selected poems of Antonio Machado*. Wesleyan University Press.

Malraux, A. (2021, June 18). *Top 30 quotes from Andre Malraux*. www.inspiringquotes.us/author/5188-andre-malraux#:~:text=%E2%80%9CThe%20first%20duty%20of%20a,anyone%20%2D%20even%20to%20himself.%E2%80%9D&text=%E2%80%9CThe%20most%20important%20thing%20in,that%20you%20are%20never%20beaten.%E2%80%9D&text=%E2%80%9CThere%20are%20not%20fifty%20ways,one%2C%20and%20that's%20to%20win

# 11 Coping

Coping mechanisms are self-regulatory processes that most clients can strengthen when they visit a human service provider. Either they do not have the internal resources to develop them or they simply have not been taught how to slowly build on their own strengths in order to generate these. Coping skills (coping strategies or coping mechanisms) are a series of tools and techniques that clients can use to help themselves handle or manage difficult emotions and sources of stress, and establish or maintain a sense of internal balance.

Coping means to invest one's own conscious effort, to solve personal and interpersonal problems, in order to minimize the impact of stress and conflict in their lives. The best way to present these coping mechanisms or skills to our clients is to use the metaphor of a tool belt. The job that a mechanic or carpenter faces will determine the type of tools needed to effectively resolve it. As clients slowly learn how to generate a set of personal tools, they will be able to keep adding layers and specific skills to enhance the methods of coping with diverse challenges in their lives. Coping strategies serve as a gauging mechanism or pressure valve that will alleviate internal emotional combustion while allowing the individual to reset and rethink clearly prior to taking action. In many ways, the counselor or human service professional adopts the role of an instructor who provides a series of techniques, skills, or mechanisms to allow the client to add them to their repertoire and apply them outside of the clinical setting. Additionally, the counselor will assist clients to unlearn a series of *negative coping strategies or skills* that they have applied for long periods of time with poor results. The job of the human service professional is to bring those to a level of personal awareness and reduce the utilization of these in the future. Some of these negative coping strategies can be over-doing certain activities like eating, drinking, or shopping to help deal with negative feelings. Then, these negative coping techniques have to be substituted with positive or more functional skills.

See also: distress tolerance, relationships, hope, and adversity

 ## Microfiction

### Downhill

Immediately after Judy's divorce things started to change rapidly. The sense of loss, grief, and anger had somewhat settled. Yet there was a sense of emptiness that was consuming her alive. All her daily routines were disrupted. The kids and the former spouse were not home and there

DOI: 10.4324/9781003145943-14

was no consensus about meals, activities, and daily chores and responsibilities. Since there was no sense of accountability, Judy stopped sweeping, vacuuming, washing dishes, feeding the pets at regular intervals and taking them out, doing laundry, preparing meals, cleaning bathrooms, and dusting. Her house looked more and more like a house on the brink of foreclosure. It appeared that it had been abandoned and used by marauders. The house was dark and pestilent. She barely made it to work on a daily basis and her coworkers were concerned about her personal hygiene. Judy stopped going out with her best friends and isolated herself as a hermit. No visits to the mall, favorite restaurants, and walks around the neighborhood and close by nature reserve. Weekdays and weekends were the same, one after the other, she simply existed. One day, her best friend came to visit her unannounced and peaked through the entrance door. "Judy, my dear friend, you need help, please let me help you deal with your situation. After all, I am your best friend." Enraged, Judy yelled at her and told her to mind her own business because she had the right to spend her life the way she wanted. Dejected, her friend stopped emailing, calling, and visiting her. Judy fell into an abyss, she was being swallowed up by the jaws of pain, isolation, and anger. She knew how best to deal with everything. Avoidance and denial. One of her strategies to deal with her current pain was to eat a gallon of ice cream at once while watching TV. Or she substituted the ice cream for a giant can of sweet popcorn. Her best friend became the TV; meaningless shows or countless hours of flipping channels became her routine. She does not remember the last time that she went out to the shopping mall or a restaurant. She felt accosted by people, irritated by the looks of others. After all, why would she care?

(*Español*)

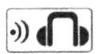 **Microficción**

### Cuesta Abajo

*Inmediatamente después del divorcio de Judy, las cosas empezaron a cambiar rápidamente. La sensación de pérdida, dolor e ira se había calmado un poco. Sin embargo, había una sensación de vacío que la consumía viva. Todas sus rutinas diarias se vieron interrumpidas. Los niños y el ex cónyuge no estaban en casa y no hubo consenso sobre las comidas, las actividades y las tareas y responsabilidades diarias. Como no tenía sentido de responsabilidad, Judy dejó de barrer, aspirar, lavar platos, alimentar a las mascotas a intervalos regulares y sacarlas, lavar la ropa, preparar comidas, limpiar baños y quitar el polvo de la casa. Su casa se parecía cada vez más a una casa al borde de la ejecución hipotecaria. Parecía que había sido abandonada y utilizada por merodeadores. La casa estaba oscura y pestilente. Apenas llegaba al trabajo todos los días y sus compañeros de trabajo estaban preocupados por su higiene personal. Judy dejó de salir con sus mejores amigas y se aisló como ermitaña. No hay visitas al centro comercial, restaurantes favoritos y caminatas por el vecindario y la reserva natural cercana. Los días laborables y los fines de semana eran iguales, uno tras otro, ella simplemente existía. Un día, su mejor amiga vino a visitarla sin previo aviso y entró por la puerta de entrada. "Judy, mi querida amiga, necesitas ayuda, por favor déjame ayudarte a lidiar con tu situación. Después de todo, soy tu mejor amiga." Enfurecida, Judy le gritó y le dijo que se ocupara de sus propios asuntos porque tenía derecho a pasar la vida como quisiera. Abatida, su amiga dejó de enviarle correos electrónicos, llamarla y visitarla. Judy cayó en un abismo, estaba siendo devorada por las mandíbulas del dolor, el aislamiento y la ira. Sabía cuál era la mejor manera de lidiar con todo. Evitación y negación. Una de sus estrategias para lidiar con su dolor actual fue comer un galón de helado de un golpe mientras miraba la televisión. O, a veces sustituía el helado por una lata gigante de palomitas de maíz dulce. Su mejor amiga se convirtió en la televisión, los programas sin sentido o las incontables horas de cambiar de canal se convirtieron en su rutina. No recuerda la última vez que salió al centro comercial o al restaurante. Se sentía acosada por la gente, irritada por las miradas de los demás. Después de todo, ¿por qué le importaría a ella?*

Author: Roberto Swazo.

*Cultural Hints*

The concept of coping, per se, might be absent in many non-Western countries, especially from an individualistic standpoint. However, coping might be part of the social fabric or culture of many individuals. For example, meals are typically consumed with family members and in large gatherings. Going for a walk in the evening with family and friends is fairly common as well as eating healthy foods. Also, depending on the religious background, congregating is part of the support network that provides strength. And, coping might be based on the idea that a higher power will provide them the strength to tolerate and manage difficult times.

**Processing questions for the clients (Preguntas de proceso para los/as clientes)**

1. Without going into deep psychological interpretations, what do you think is going on with Judy? (*Sin entrar en interpretaciones psicológicas profundas, ¿qué crees que está pasando con Judy?*)
2. Make a list of the negative coping strategies that Judy is using on a daily basis. And, what strategies would you use to counter these? Discuss. (*Haz una lista de las estrategias de manejo negativas que Judy utiliza a diario. ¿Y qué estrategias utilizarías para contrarrestarlas? Discutir.*)
3. At what point in your life have you done things similar to Judy in order to cope with your challenging moments? Have you overcome these or have you relapsed? Elaborate. (*¿En qué momento de tu vida has hecho cosas similares a las de Judy para hacer frente a tus momentos difíciles? ¿Los has superado o has recaído? Elaborar.*)

*Table 11.1* Common Grief-Related Concerns and Coping Skill Exploration

| Problem | Coping skill | Comments |
| --- | --- | --- |
| Some type of fear is blocking your progress (i.e., fear of heights, animals, insects, crowds) [*Algún tipo de miedo está bloqueando tu progreso (es decir, miedo a las alturas, animales, insectos, multitudes)*] | | |

*(Continued)*

*Table 11.1* (Continued)

| Problem | Coping skill | Comments |
|---|---|---|
| High levels of stress (*Altos niveles de estrés*) | | |
| Personal friends are sabotaging your life (*Los amigos personales están saboteando tu vida*) | | |
| The routine is taking the best out of you (*La rutina está sacando lo mejor de ti*) | | |
| You feel mentally, psychologically, and emotionally exhausted and unable to keep going on (*La rutina está sacando lo mejor de ti*) | | |
| You feel as if your life has lost meaning (*Sientes como si tu vida hubiera perdido sentido*) | | |
| You made a series of bad decisions that affected other people (*Tomaste una serie de malas decisiones que afectaron a otras personas*) | | |
| A romantic, personal, or social relationship ended (*Una relación romántica, personal o social terminó*) | | |
| You are physically and emotionally unhealthy (*No tienes salud física y emocional*) | | |
| Your personal finances are out of control (*Tus finanzas personales están fuera de control*) | | |
| Your professional career is not advancing and you feel stuck (*Tu carrera profesional no avanza y te sientes estancado*) | | |
| A person/s have criticized you and you feel offended (*Una persona te ha criticado y te sientes ofendido*) | | |

| Problem | Coping skill | Comments |
|---|---|---|
| You have not been able to reach your personal or professional goals<br>(*No has podido alcanzar tus objetivos personales o profesionales*) | | |
| You feel confused about many issues and unable to make a decision<br>(*Te sientes confundido por muchos problemas y no puedes tomar una decisión*) | | |
| Your past is always present and you are unable to shake it off<br>(*Tu pasado siempre está presente y no puedes deshacerte de él*) | | |
| You cannot stop grieving<br>(*No puedes dejar de llorar*) | | |

 **Sayings (*dichos*)**

 *Saying #1*

"Money and possessions will not make you happy and healthy if you are enslaved by them."
*"El dinero y las posesiones no te harán feliz ni saludable si te esclavizan."*

Author: Unknown. Popular Arab saying (A. Faheem, personal communication, May 21, 2018).

**Processing questions for the clients (Preguntas de proceso para los/as clientes)**

1. From the picture that follows, what happens when both of our arms are holding money and possessions? Are there any extra arms to give a hug, extend a helping hand, or fix something that needs to be rearranged? Explain. (*De la siguiente imagen, ¿qué sucede cuando ambos brazos sostienen dinero y posesiones? ¿Hay brazos adicionales para dar un abrazo, extender una mano amiga o arreglar algo que necesita ser reorganizado? Explicar.*)

2. If you want to find a balance between achieving your goals and acquiring personal possessions, it is important to remember that after all the following are simple ways to keep you grounded and real: (*Si deseas encontrar un equilibrio entre el logro de tus metas y la adquisición de posesiones personales, es importante recordar que, después de todo, las siguientes son formas sencillas de mantenerse firme y real:*)

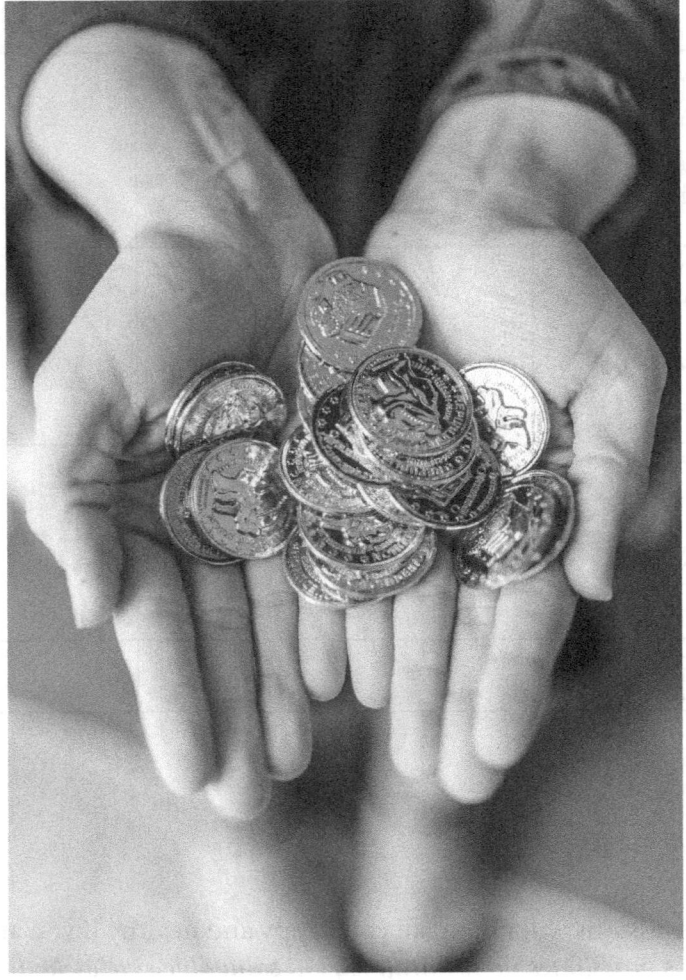

*Figure 11.1*  Woman Holding Golden Coins in Her Open Hands

- ride a bicycle.
- feed the ducks, birds, squirrels, or local wildlife and enjoy their interactions.
- color in a color book.
- memorize a poem, play, or song that serves as an inspiration.
- stretch on the ground for 20–25 minutes.
- search for ridiculous things on the Internet that make you laugh.
- watch fish either in a tank, beach, lake, or river.
- make a CD/playlist of your favorite songs and make sure that you listen to them frequently.
- help a friend or relative plan a wedding/prom/other event.
- plant some seeds and make sure that you take care of them.
- try to make as many words out of your full name as possible and write them down.
- sort through/edit your pictures and create categories and comments by them.
- give yourself a facial or get an appointment for a massage.
- start collecting something.

- clean up trash at your local park and do not tell anyone about it.
- text or call an old friend that you have not talked to in a long time.
- write yourself an "I love you because . . ." letter.
- look up new words and use them, be it in your native language or a different one.
- rearrange the furniture of your house or apartment.
- write a letter to someone that you may never send, keep it with you and decide when it needs to be discarded.
- smile at five people and say hello to them.
- play with your little brother/sister/niece/nephew and turn off your phone while doing this.
- go for a walk (with or without a friend) and don't bring your phone.
- put a puzzle together while having nice background music.

**(Spanish list)**

- *Montar en bicicleta.*
- *Alimenta a los patos, pájaros, ardillas, o vida salvaje local y disfrutar de sus interacciones.*
- *Colorea un libro de colores.*
- *Memoriza un poema, obra de teatro o canción que te sirva de inspiración.*
- *Estírate en el suelo durante 20–25 minutos.*
- *Busca cosas ridículas en Internet que te hagan reír.*
- *Observa peces en un tanque, playa, lago o río.*
- *Haz un CD/lista de reproducción de tus canciones favoritas y asegúrate de escucharlas con frecuencia.*
- *Ayuda a un amigo o familiar a planificar la boda, el baile de graduación u otro evento.*
- *Planta algunas semillas y asegúrate de cuidarlas.*
- *Trata de hacer la mayor cantidad posible de palabras con tu nombre completo y escríbelas.*
- *Ordena/edita tus imágenes y crea categorías y comentarios para ellas.*
- *Regálate un facial o pide una cita para un masaje.*
- *Empieza a coleccionar algo.*
- *Limpia la basura en tu parque local y no se lo cuentes a nadie.*
- *Envía un mensaje de texto o llama a un viejo amigo con el que no has hablado en mucho tiempo.*
- *Escríbete una carta de "Te amo porque . . . "*
- *Busca nuevas palabras y úsalas, ya sea en tu idioma nativo o en uno diferente.*
- *Reorganiza los muebles de tu casa o apartamento.*
- *Escribe una carta a alguien que quizás nunca envíes, guárdala y decide cuándo debes desecharla.*
- *Sonría a cinco personas y salúdalas.*
- *Juega con tu hermano pequeño/hermana/sobrina/sobrino y apaga tu teléfono mientras haces esto.*
- *Sal a caminar (con o sin un amigo) y no traigas tu teléfono.*
- *Arma un rompecabezas mientras tiene una buena música de fondo.*

3. Based on the stress generated by making money and acquiring possessions, complete the following incomplete sentences: (*Con base en el estrés que genera ganar dinero y adquirir posesiones, completa las siguientes oraciones incompletas:*)

- I promise that I will_____. (*Prometo que _____.*)
- I recognize that I have issues with_____. (*Reconozco que tengo problemas con _____.*)
- I am unable to manage_____ when_____. (*No puedo manejar _____ cuando _____.*)
- I cannot deal with_____. (*No puedo lidiar con _____.*)
- I will not let_____ ruin my life. (*No dejaré que _____ arruine mi vida.*)
- I have noticed that I have changed in the following ways_____, _____, _____, etc. (*He notado que he cambiado de las siguientes formas _____, _____, _____, etc.*)
- If I could change something about what I am doing right now, I would change_____. (*Si pudiera cambiar algo sobre lo que estoy haciendo ahora mismo, cambiaría _____.*)
- Those around me tell me that my behavior is_____. (*Los que me rodean me dicen que mi comportamiento es _____.*)

## Saying #2

"The others are not the problem but the way your eyes see them."
   "*Los otros no son el problema, sino la forma en que los ven tus ojos.*"

Author: Unknown. Popular Turkish saying (B. Özdemir, personal communication, January 1, 2019).

## Processing questions for the clients (Preguntas de proceso para los/as clientes)

1. What is your personal definition of a problem? Explain. (*¿Cuál es tu definición personal de un problema? Explicar.*)
2. Based on your personal experiences, have your problems been similar to those of others? If not, how so? (*Según tus experiencias personales, ¿tus problemas han sido similares a los de los demás? Si no es así, ¿cómo es eso?*)
3. How would you cope with the following problems in life? (*¿Cómo afrontarías los siguientes problemas en la vida?*)

## Quotes

## Quote #1

"One of life's best coping mechanisms is to know the difference between an inconvenience and a problem."
   "*Uno de los mejores mecanismos de manejo en la vida es saber la diferencia entre un inconveniente y un problema.*"

Author: Robert Fulghum (2010). He is an American author and Unitarian Universalist minister.

 **Processing questions for the clients (Preguntas de proceso para los/as clientes)**

1. Rank the following as inconveniences or problems (I or P): [*Clasifica los siguientes como inconvenientes o problemas (I o P):*]

*Table 11.2* Problem or Inconvenience Activity Table

| | Inconvenience or problem (*Inconveniencia o problema*) (I or P) | What makes you think that this is an inconvenience or a problem? Explain. (*¿Qué te hace pensar que esto es un inconveniente o un problema? Explicar.*) |
|---|---|---|
| Unraveling your headphones (*Desenredar tus auriculares*) | | |
| Being the first at a social gathering and feeling obligated to wait for those who come late (*Ser el primero en una reunión social y sentirse obligado a esperar a los que llegan tarde*) | | |
| Running out of phone battery in a public place and being unable to recharge it (*Quedarse sin batería del teléfono en un lugar público y no poder recargarla*) | | |
| Having to enter captcha or clicking on pictures to prove your identity on your computer or phone (*Tener que ingresar captcha o hacer clic en las imágenes para demostrar tu identidad en tu computadora o teléfono*) | | |
| Getting a slightly different haircut than you had imagined (*Recibir un corte de pelo ligeramente diferente al que habías imaginado*) | | |
| Having to use a public toilet (*Tener que usar un baño público*) | | |
| Being locked out of your personal account for using the wrong password several times (*Ser bloqueado de tu cuenta personal por usar la contraseña incorrecta varias veces*) | | |

*(Continued)*

*Table 11.2* (Continued)

| | Inconvenience or problem (*Inconveniencia o problema*) (I or P) | What makes you think that this is an inconvenience or a problem? Explain. (*¿Qué te hace pensar que esto es un inconveniente o un problema? Explicar.*) |
|---|---|---|
| Forgetting to bring your raincoat or umbrella and getting wet (*Olvidar traer tu impermeable o paraguas y mojarte*) | | |
| Your Internet is down for a few minutes (*Tu conexión a la Internet está inactiva durante unos minutos*) | | |
| Having to stand up and put your meal plate because your remote control is not working well (*Tener que levantarse y guardar tu plato de comida porque tu control remoto no funciona bien*) | | |
| Not having enough milk or yogurt in the morning while getting ready to eat breakfast (*No tener suficiente leche o yogur por la mañana mientras te preparas para desayunar*) | | |
| Barely missing your train or bus as you were approaching it (*Apenas pierdes el tren o el autobús cuando te acercabas al mismo*) | | |
| Having to wake up to pee after being cozy in bed (*Tener que despertarse para orinar después de estar cómodo en la cama*) | | |
| Stepping on a wet patch at home and getting your socks wet (you realize that your dog had an accident) [*Pisar una mancha húmeda en casa y mojarse los calcetines (te das cuenta de que tu perro tuvo un accidente)*] | | |
| Someone ate the leftovers in the fridge that you were saving for today's dinner (*Alguien se comió las sobras en el refrigerador que estabas guardando para la cena de hoy*) | | |

2. **Miracle question:** If you had a chance to make your problems disappear, which problems would these be? List and explain. And, if you could add intuitively to your personal assets a number of coping strategies, what would these be? List and explain. (***Pregunta milagrosa:*** *si tuvieras la oportunidad de hacer desaparecer tus problemas, ¿cuáles serían? Enumere y explique. Y, si pudieras agregar intuitivamente a tus activos personales una serie de estrategias de manejo, ¿cuáles serían? Enumere y explique.*)

3. **Flagging the Minefield technique:** From the exercises and strategies provided in this section, what has worked best for you? What have you learned from these and what would you do differently if you had a chance to apply any of these coping strategies again? Elaborate. (***La técnica de marcar el campo minado:*** *De los ejercicios y estrategias proporcionados en esta sección, ¿qué ha funcionado mejor para ti? ¿Qué has aprendido de ellos y qué harías de manera diferente si tuvieras la oportunidad de aplicar alguna de estas estrategias de manejo nuevamente? Elaborar.*)

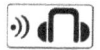

### Quote #2

"We have two strategies for coping; the way of avoidance or the way of attention."
*"Tenemos dos estrategias de manejo; la forma de evitación o la forma de atención."*

Author: Marilyn Ferguson (2009). She was an American author, editor, and public speaker.

### Processing questions for the clients (Preguntas de proceso para los/as clientes)

1. Create a personal/historical map of specific challenging times that have impacted your life and proved to be difficult for you. For instance, moving to a new school, dealing with parents' divorce, losing a loved one, moving to a new state or country, dealing with a medical diagnosis, helping a significant other with an addiction, etc. Then, generate a list of the coping strategies you used to deal with these events. Rank these in order of positive impact and negative impact or outcome. Finally, determine if there have been any overlapping themes or repetitions of using negative coping strategies. What can be changed? Discuss.

   (*Crea un mapa personal/histórico de momentos difíciles específicos que han impactado tu vida y han demostrado ser difíciles para ti. Por ejemplo, mudarse a una nueva escuela, lidiar con el divorcio de los padres, perder a un ser querido, mudarse a un nuevo estado o país, lidiar con un diagnóstico médico, ayudar a una pareja con una adicción, etc. Luego, genera una lista de las estrategias de manejo que utilizaste para lidiar con estos eventos. Clasifícalos en orden de impacto positivo e impacto o resultado negativo. Finalmente, determina si ha habido temas superpuestos o repeticiones del uso de estrategias de manejo negativas. ¿Qué se puede cambiar? Discutir.*)

2. How many times have you used the following negative coping strategies in your life? Circle the ones that you use the most and determine how these can be turned into positive coping strategies.

   (*¿Cuántas veces has utilizado las siguientes estrategias de manejo negativas en su vida? Encierra en un círculo las que más utilizas y determina cómo se pueden convertir en estrategias de manejo positivas.*)

Diversions or distractions (*Desviaciones o distracciones*)

- procrastination. (*Dilación.*)
- abusing drugs or alcohol. (*Abusar de drogas o alcohol.*)
- wasting time on unimportant tasks. (*Perder tiempo en tareas sin importancia.*)

Interpersonal, relational, or social (*Interpersonal, relacional o social*)

- blaming. (*Culpar.*)
- isolating/withdrawing. (*Aislarse/retirarse.*)
- mean or hostile joking. (*Bromas malas u hostiles.*)
- gossiping. (*Chismes.*)
- criticizing others. (*Criticar a los demás.*)
- manipulating others. (*Manipular a otros.*)
- refusing help from others. (*Rechazar la ayuda de otros.*)
- lying to others. (*Mentir a los demás.*)
- sabotaging plans. (*Auto sabotear tus planes.*)
- being late to appointments. (*Llegar tarde a las citas.*)
- provoking violence from others. (*Provocar la violencia de otros.*)
- enabling others to take advantage of you. (*Permitir que otros se aprovechen de ti.*)

3. Based on the quote, what has prompted you to avoid a problem as opposed to being attentive to it? And, for how long have you avoided important issues that need to be addressed? List the feelings of relief once these avoided issues have been resolved. Elaborate on your answers. (*Según la cita, ¿qué te ha llevado a evitar un problema en lugar de estar atento a él? Y, ¿durante cuánto tiempo has evitado cuestiones importantes que deben abordarse? Enumera los sentimientos de alivio una vez que se hayan resuelto estos problemas evitados. Desarrolla tus respuestas.*)

### Quote #3

"Problems are not the problem; coping is the problem."
"*Los problemas no son el problema; manejarlos es el problema.*"

Author: Virginia Satir. She was an influential American author and psychotherapist, recognized for her approach to family therapy (Baldwin et al., 1983).

### Processing questions for the clients (Preguntas de proceso para los/as clientes)

1. What is the meaning of this quote? What is the difference between a subjective and objective perspective of an event? Do you see everything as a problem or a challenge and opportunity to grow as a professional, parent, friend, lover, etc.? (*¿Cuál es el significado de esta cita? ¿Cuál es la diferencia entre una perspectiva subjetiva y objetiva de un evento? ¿Ves todo como un problema o como un desafío y una oportunidad para crecer como profesional, padre, amigo, amante, etc.?*)

2. Following the theme of the quote, how many times have you coped by doing the following? Create a counter positive strategy for the ones selected. (*Siguiendo el tema de la cita, ¿cuántas veces has manejado los siguientes de la siguiente manera? Crea una estrategia contra-positiva para los seleccionados.*)

**Cognitive (mind/thinking process)** [*Cognitivo (Proceso mental/pensamiento)*]

- denying any problem. (*Negando cualquier problema.*)
- stubbornness/inflexibility. (*Terquedad/inflexibilidad.*)
- all or nothing/black or white thinking. (*Todo o nada/pensamiento en blanco o negro.*)
- catastrophizing. (*Catastrofizar.*)
- overgeneralizing. (*Sobregeneralizar.*)

**Intrapersonal (internal process)** [(*Intrapersonal (proceso interno)*)]

- making fun of yourself. (*Burlarte de ti mismo.*)
- self-sabotaging behaviors. (*Comportamientos de autosabotaje.*)
- blaming yourself. (*Culparte a ti mismo.*)

3. Make copies of the table that follows and determine which of these positive coping strategies can be used during moments of stress be they internal or external during the next month: (*Haz copias de la tabla a continuación y determina cuáles de estas estrategias de manejo positivas se pueden usar durante los momentos de estrés, ya sean internos o externos, durante el próximo mes:*)

*Table 11.3* Stressors and Potential Corresponding Coping Strategies

| Stressor (*Estresante*) | Coping strategy (*Estrategia de manejo*) | Comments (*Comentarios*) |
| --- | --- | --- |
| | Exercise (running, walking, etc.) [*Ejercicio (correr, caminar, etc.)*] | |
| | Do schoolwork (*Hacer el trabajo escolar*) | |
| | Play a musical instrument (*Tocar un instrumento musical*) | |
| | Paint your nails, do your make-up or hair (*Pintarte tus uñas, maquillarte o peinarte*) | |
| | Sing (*Cantar*) | |
| | Read a good book (*Leer un buen libro*) | |
| | Study las estrellas (*Observar el firmamento/estrellas*) | |
| | Punch a punching bag (*Golpear un saco de boxeo*) | |

(Continued)

*Table 11.2* (Continued)

| Stressor (*Estresante*) | Coping strategy (*Estrategia de manejo*) | Comments (*Comentarios*) |
|---|---|---|
| | Let yourself cry and take a nap (only if you are tired) [*Llorar y toma una siesta (solo si estás cansado)*] | |
| | Take a hot shower or relaxing bath (*Toma una ducha caliente o un baño relajante*) | |
| | Play with a pet (*Jugar con una mascota*) | |
| | Go shopping (*Ir de compras*) | |
| | Clean something (*Limpiar algo*) | |
| | Knit or sew (*Tejer o coser*) | |
| | Put on fake tattoos (*Ponerte tatuajes falsos*) | |
| | Write (poetry, stories, journal) [*Escribir (poesía, cuentos, diario)*] | |
| | Scribble/doodle on paper (*Hacer garabatos en un papel*) | |
| | Be with other people (*Compartir con otras personas*) | |
| | Watch a favorite TV show (*Ver tu programa favorito de la TV*) | |
| | Post on web boards, and answer others' posts (*Publica en foros web y responde a las publicaciones de otros*) | |
| | Go see a movie (*Ve a ver una película*) | |
| | Do a word search or crossword (*Hacer una búsqueda de palabras o un crucigrama*) | |

## References

Baldwin, M., Satir, V., & Blockley, R. (1983). *Satir step by step: A guide to creating change in families.* Science and Behavior Books, p. 166.

Ferguson, M. (2009). *The aquarian conspiracy: Personal and social transformation in our time.* Jeremy P. Tarcher/Penguin, p. 76.

Fulghum, R. (2010). *Uh-Oh: Some observations from both sides of the refrigerator door.* Random House Publishing Group, p. 146.

# 12 Distress Tolerance

Coping with and tolerating the spectrum of emotion is a universal human experience. Emotion and distress, however, are experienced differently by each person. Tolerating distress includes the ways in which individuals manage real or perceived emotional distress or tension. Stressors can range from daily hassles to more complex traumas or losses. Clients who are able to increase their tolerance or coping skills to deal with these daily events are less likely to become overwhelmed, to engage in self-harming or destructive behavior, and to experience less mental health impacts, as a result.

Helping clients distinguish between the value of their emotions and emotions that can feel debilitating or paralyzing can help clients harness emotions and utilize them in ways that are effective and productive. Fear, for example, is a present experience and serves to prepare one for an immediate threat, while anxiety is a future focused event that includes thoughts and physiological responses to what *could* happen in the future. Anxiety and worry may also have useful features, such as preparing for the future, or less adaptive features, such as ruminating and obsessing over future outcomes. Similarly, anger can serve as an indicator of an injustice and move individuals toward change, or it can evolve into bitterness, apathy, and hopelessness. When assessing each client's level of distress, it is critical to assess for safety (e.g., self-harming behaviors or risk to self or others), which will guide what activities may be appropriate to utilize. For example, individuals who are at risk for self-harm or who have a history of self-harm may benefit from activities that utilize distraction, grounding, or replacement behaviors, rather than activities that lead to a focusing on the distressing emotion(s).

See also: coping, adversity, grief and loss, and hope

##  Cultural Hints

Emotional distress, while universal, varies in meaning, value, and purpose across cultures. Eastern cultures may view suffering and pain as a necessary and acceptable part of existence, whereas Western cultures may go to great lengths to avoid discomfort and distress. Additionally, avoidance measures may be utilized in order to project more socially acceptable markers of happiness. Similarly, religious themes, such as an understanding of suffering or distress as a consequence of sin, process of cultivating faith or experiencing personal growth may shift the experience and perception of emotional pain. Identifying the value and meaning of each client's experience can prevent pathologizing behavior and conceptualization.

DOI: 10.4324/9781003145943-15

**Microfiction**

### The Cloak

My shoulders and back ache, my legs strain under the pressure, and my arms are sluggish in their movement. I am suffocating in this cloak, desperation taking over as I negotiate my breaths. *Breathe! Fight!* I can barely stand to exist in it, and yet, I can't remove the item. My fingers have stopped clawing at the clasps, as the realization accelerates the pounding in my chest and I feel trapped, my garment blazing in furious shades of orange, red, purple, and black. Rough spikes protrude from the fabric and scratch my skin. The heat building underneath the cloak brings an angry flush to my face, as beads of sweat pool at my temples. *I'm trapped. I am trapped. I'm suffocating.* An anguished shout is ripped from my lungs, the scream becoming less like a voice, and more like a rasp. The weight in the cloth becomes overwhelming, and I slump to the ground in defeat. *I'm suffocating.* Droplets of sweat begin to mix with my tears, as I allow my forehead to touch the ground. The feeling of cool earth on my face is a shock, and extracts another sharp breath. I lay here. And I stay this way. And the forest is none the wiser.

In my periphery, I am aware that the blinding colors of my cloak have melted into intense swirls of black, purples, and blues, the reds, oranges, and yellows dissolving into the mix. The movement of colors reluctantly slows down, as the hours pass me by, and the fabric's surface smooths. My tears nearly dry, and my chest feels hollow. A slower movement mesmerizes me, and I angle my chin to the side to widen my view. A sleepy series of ripples undulates between soft greens and light blues across my arms, back, and legs, where the cloak has covered me. A calm after the storm.

In moving to lift my head from its bowed position on the ground, I notice that my arms come easily with the movement. There is a lightness to the cloak that wasn't present before; an emptying that took place, while I had sheltered from my storm.

I press myself from the ground, feeling new aches and tensions that had settled over the last several hours, and stumble back to my village in search of the one who gave me this cloak.

When I arrived, I saw the old man. His detail lost in my hazy gaze, but his shape and sound clear. "Why did you give me this cloak?! Why do you make me wear it?" I cry, hoarsely.

He regards me tenderly. His eyes are unfazed by my appearance, so similar to the look that he gave me this morning, when he draped me with the warm fabric. "It is not that I made you wear it. It is that you are always wearing it. The cloak simply illustrates what is already underneath. You carry these feelings with you always. Did you check the inner pockets of your cloak, to see the burdens that weigh on you, but are hidden from others? Did you feel the ways in which your anger can cut and scrape you and others? And yet, these experiences are always yours. You were capable of waiting out the tempest, even when it felt unlikely."

*(Español)*

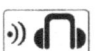 **Microficción**

### El Manto

*Me duelen los hombros y la espalda, mis piernas se tensan bajo la presión y mis brazos se mueven con lentitud. Me ahogo en esta capa, la desesperación se apodera de mí mientras reprimo mis respiraciones. ¡Respirar! ¡Lucha! Apenas puedo soportar existir en él y, sin embargo, no puedo eliminar el elemento. Mis dedos han dejado de arañar los broches, ya que la comprensión acelera los latidos en mi pecho y me siento atrapada, mi prenda resplandece en furiosos tonos de naranja, rojo, morado y negro. Las puntas ásperas sobresalen de la tela y me raspan la piel. El calor que se acumula debajo de la capa me provoca un rubor de ira en la cara, mientras gotas de sudor se acumulan en mis sienes. Estoy atrapado. Estoy atrapado. Me estoy sofocando. Un grito de angustia sale de mis pulmones, el grito se vuelve menos como una voz y más como un chirrido. El peso de la tela se vuelve abrumador y caigo al suelo derrotado.*

*Me estoy sofocando. Las gotas de sudor comienzan a mezclarse con mis lágrimas, mientras dejo que mi frente toque el suelo. La sensación de tierra fría en mi rostro es un shock, y me extrae otro aliento agudo. Me acuesto aquí. Y me quedo así. Y el bosque no se da cuenta.*

*En mi periferia, soy consciente de que los colores cegadores de mi manto se han fundido en intensos remolinos de negros, púrpuras y azules, rojos, naranjas y amarillos, disolviéndose en la mezcla. El movimiento de los colores se ralentiza a regañadientes, a medida que pasan las horas y la superficie de la tela se suaviza. Mis lágrimas casi se secan y mi pecho se siente vacío. Un movimiento más lento me hipnotiza, e inclino la barbilla hacia un lado para ampliar mi vista. Una serie de ondas somnolientas ondulan entre verdes suaves y azules claros en mis brazos, espalda y piernas, donde la capa me ha cubierto. Una calma después de la tormenta.*

*Al moverme para levantar la cabeza de su posición inclinada en el suelo, noto que mis brazos se aflojan fácilmente con el movimiento. Hay una ligereza en la capa que no estaba presente antes; un vaciamiento que tuvo lugar, mientras me había resguardado de mi tormenta. Me presiono desde el suelo, sintiendo nuevos dolores y tensiones que se han asentado durante las últimas horas, y vuelvo a mi aldea a trompicones en busca de quien me dio esta capa.*

*Cuando llegué, vi al anciano. Su detalle se perdió en mi mirada nebulosa, pero su forma y su sonido son claros. "¡¿Por qué me diste esta capa?! ¿Por qué me obligas a usarlo?" Lloro roncamente.*

*Me mira con ternura. Sus ojos no se inmutan por mi apariencia, tan similar a la mirada que me dio esta mañana, cuando me cubrió con la cálida tela. "No es que yo te obligué a usarlo. Es que siempre lo llevas puesto. La capa simplemente ilustra lo que ya está debajo. Siempre llevas estos sentimientos contigo. ¿Revisaste los bolsillos interiores de tu manto para ver las cargas que pesan sobre ti, pero que están ocultas a los demás? ¿Sintió las formas en que su ira puede cortarlo y rasparlo a usted y a los demás? Y, sin embargo, estas experiencias son siempre tuyas. Fuiste capaz de esperar a que pasara la tempestad, incluso cuando parecía poco probable."*

Author: Noelany Pelc.

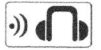 **Processing questions for the clients (Preguntas de proceso para los/as clientes)**

1. What did the cloak represent in this story? (*¿Qué representa la capa en esta historia?*)

2. In your opinion, what did the older man know, that he wanted to teach the main character? What lessons are you hoping to learn about your distressing experiences? (*En tu opinión, ¿qué sabía el hombre mayor, que quería enseñarle al personaje principal? ¿Qué lecciones espera aprender acerca de sus angustiantes experiencias?*)

3. What would your cloak represent? What colors, textures, and images would be represented during difficult moments for you? What is held in your pockets that others don't know? (*¿Qué representaría tu manto? ¿Qué colores, texturas e imágenes se representarían durante los momentos difíciles para ti? ¿Qué tienes en los bolsillos que otros no saben?*)

4. What does the transition of your emotions look like? Imagine the transition of intense and bright emotions, to the more relaxed and calm emotions. How does this process generally take place? What do you do in order to ride out your storms? (*¿Cómo se ve la transición de tus emociones? Imagínate la transición de emociones intensas y brillantes a más de las emociones más relajadas y tranquilas. ¿Cómo se lleva a cabo este proceso en general? ¿Qué haces para capear tus tormentas?*)

5. There are numerous effective interventions for coping with distress. Visit the Dialectical Behavior Therapy webpage, and identify two or three primary ways in which you could cope with distress. The authors offer ten different approaches, each with examples and skills to practice. Look for concrete ideas that you can practice in advance and successfully implement when you are in distress. (*Existen numerosas intervenciones eficaces para afrontar la angustia. Visita la página web de Terapia de comportamiento dialéctico e identifica dos o tres formas principales en las que podrías afrontar la angustia. Los autores ofrecen diez enfoques diferentes, cada uno con ejemplos y habilidades para practicar. Busca ideas concretas que puedas practicar de antemano e implementar con éxito cuando te encuentres en peligro.*)

Link in English: https://dialecticalbehaviortherapy.com/distress-tolerance/
Resources in Spanish: www.dbtselfhelp.com/

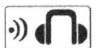 **Sayings (*dichos*)**

 *Saying #1*

"Anger has no eyes."
   "*La ira no tiene ojos.*"

Author: Unknown. Hindi Proverb (2021).

**Processing questions for the clients (Preguntas de proceso para los/as clientes)**

1. How does your anger blind you? What other senses and experiences are altered in your anger? (*¿Cómo te ciega tu ira? ¿Qué otros sentidos y experiencias se alteran en tu ira?*)

2. If anger were to add other feelings, how does anger amplify or dampen your other emotions? Make a list of the emotions that often accompany your anger, or that you might experience along with anger. Draw them as dials, where you can indicate how strongly you typically experience each emotion, and the influence of anger on each dial. What patterns emerge for you? (*Si la ira agregara otros sentimientos, ¿cómo la ira amplifica o amortigua tus otras emociones? Haz una lista de las emociones que a menudo acompañan a tu enojo, o que podrías experimentar junto con el enojo. Dibujarlos como un selector, donde puedes indicar con qué intensidad experimenta cada emoción y la influencia de la ira en cada selector. ¿Qué patrones surgen para ti?*)

3. If you were a character in a story and were blinded by anger, what would an adjustment to your vision show you about your story context that you cannot yet see? (*Si fueras un*

personaje de una historia y estuvieras cegado por la ira, ¿qué te mostraría un ajuste en tu visión sobre el contexto de tu historia que aún no puedes ver?)

 *Saying #2*

"When the winds of change blow, some people build walls and others build windmills."
   "*Cuando soplan los vientos del cambio, algunas personas construyen muros y otras construyen molinos de viento.*"

Author: Unknown. Chinese Proverb (2021).

 **Processing questions for the clients (Preguntas de proceso para los/as clientes)**

1.  What does this saying mean to you? (*¿Qué significa este dicho para ti?*)
2.  In what moments in your life have you built walls? When have you chosen to build windmills? (*¿En qué momentos de tu vida has construido muros? ¿Cuándo has elegido construir molinos de viento?*)
3.  How would an outsider describe a windmill for your current situation? How would it function? How would it operate? What would it do for you? (*¿Cómo describiría un forastero un molino de viento en tu situación actual? ¿Cómo funciona el mismo? ¿Cómo funcionaría para ti?*)
4.  If you were to repurpose a wall into a windmill today, what would it require you to let go of? (*Si tuvieras que reutilizar una pared en un molino de viento hoy, ¿qué se requeriría que la soltaras?*)
5.  Write a journal entry describing the process of repurposing the wall, including: (*Escribe una entrada de diario que describa el proceso de reutilización del muro, que incluya:*)

    a.  How the wall has served you. (*Cómo te ha servido el muro.*)
    b.  Describe how and why you erected it, in the first place. (*Describe cómo y por qué lo erigiste, en primer lugar.*)
    c.  Identify and explain the feelings that come up when you think about dismantling your wall. (*Identifica y explica los sentimientos que surgen cuando piensas en desmantelar tu muro.*)
    d.  Discuss the prospect of building a windmill. What offers you the most hope, peace, and enthusiasm about constructing a windmill? Spend some time exploring these feelings and what they might mean for the future. (*Analice la posibilidad de construir un molino de viento. ¿Qué te ofrece más esperanza, paz y entusiasmo sobre la construcción de un molino de viento? Dedica algún tiempo a explorar estos sentimientos y lo que podrían significar para el futuro.*)
    e.  Finally, reflect on the time that it takes to undertake a building project. What does this translate to your own life? (*Por último, reflexiona sobre el tiempo que lleva emprender un proyecto de edificación. ¿Qué se traduce esto en tu propia vida?*)
    f.  Identify a compassionate thought about the effort and time that it takes to make even welcome improvements. (*Identifica un pensamiento compasivo sobre el esfuerzo y el tiempo que se necesita para hacer mejoras necesarias.*)

·)) 🎧  *Saying #3*

"Worry gives a small thing a big shadow."
   "La preocupación le da a una cosa pequeña una gran sombra."

Author: Unknown. Swedish Proverb (Holmes, 2021, p. 50).

·)) 🎧  **Processing questions for the clients (Preguntas de proceso para los/as clientes)**

1. What shadows loom over your life? (*¿Qué sombras se ciernen sobre tu vida?*)
2. When do these shadows tend to seem the largest? (*¿Cuándo tienden a parecer más grandes estas sombras?*)
3. If you had a recipe, what ingredients make up your worry? What are the proportions of each ingredient? (*Si tuvieras una receta, ¿qué ingredientes te preocupan? ¿Cuáles son las proporciones de cada ingrediente?*)
4. If available, find an open area of concrete, sidewalk, grass, or space on the floor. (*Si está disponible, busca un área abierta de concreto, acera, césped o espacio en el piso.*)

   a. Using any time of medium available to you (e.g., chalk, tape, pencil, marker, paint), draw an outline of yourself on the ground. (*Utilizando cualquier medio disponible para usted (por ejemplo, tiza, cinta adhesiva, lápiz, marcador, pintura), dibuja un contorno de tí mismo en el suelo.*)
   b. Next, illustrate the shadows that are currently looming over you, and draw them to size. This means drawing the shadows to the size that they currently feel, and indicating the ingredients and proportions of your worry. (*A continuación, ilustra las sombras que se ciernen sobre ti y dibújalas a su tamaño natural. Esto significa dibujar las sombras al tamaño que sienten actualmente e indicar los ingredientes y las proporciones de su preocupación.*)
   c. Now, take some time to identify that these worries exist for you and draw your attention to the present moment. (*Ahora, tómate un tiempo para identificar que estas preocupaciones existen para ti y dirige tu atención al momento presente.*)

5. What can you do to improve this moment in time? (*¿Qué puedes hacer para mejorar este momento en el tiempo?*)

   a. "What if" something positive were to happen right now? What could go well? What could make these worries slightly smaller? (*¿Y si algo positivo sucediera ahora mismo? ¿Qué podría salir bien? ¿Qué podría hacer que estas preocupaciones sean un poco menores?*)
   b. "What if" your concern(s) worked out better than you expected? "What if" your worst case scenarios do not occur? (*¿Y si tu (s) inquietud (s) funcionó mejor de lo que esperabas? "¿Qué pasa si" los peores escenarios posibles no ocurren?*)
   c. Re-draw (in a different color or medium) how your worries might change. Alter the size, composition, and proportion of each one, should there be more positive outcomes. (*Vuelve a dibujar (en un color o medio diferente), cómo podrían cambiar tus preocupaciones. Modifica el tamaño, la composición y la proporción de cada uno, en caso de que haya resultados más positivos.*)

6. "What if" you would move around the day allowing this shadow to exist, but having the power to shrink it? (*¿Y si te movieras por el día permitiendo que esta sombra exista, pero teniendo el poder de encogerla?*)

## Quotes

 *Quote #1*

"May the stars carry your sadness away, May the flowers fill your heart with beauty, May hope forever wipe away your tears, And, above all, may silence make you strong."
   *"Que las estrellas se lleven tu tristeza, que las flores llenen de belleza tu corazón, que la esperanza para siempre enjugue tus lágrimas y, sobre todo, que el silencio te haga fuerte".*

Author: Chief Dan George was Chief of the Tsleil-Waututh First Nation in North Vancouver, Canada (2021).

 **Processing questions for the clients (Preguntas de proceso para los/as clientes)**

1. How do you feel, as you read this quote? Is there a particular element that appeals to you most? Explain. (*¿Cómo te sientes al leer esta cita? ¿Hay algún elemento en particular que te atraiga más? Explicar.*)
2. Take a moment to find a quiet place where you can reflect. Identify a couple of items. What elements in nature offer you the most comfort? What experiences in your past have prompted a sense of calm, joy, peace, and/or stability? (*Tómate un momento para encontrar un lugar tranquilo donde puedas reflexionar. Identifica un par de elementos. ¿Qué elementos de la naturaleza te ofrecen más comodidad? ¿Qué experiencias en tu pasado te han provocado una sensación de calma, alegría, paz y/o estabilidad?*)
3. Similarly, what, in your environment, produces a different feeling than the uncomfortable one you are experiencing? What can you do to bring about this feeling? (*De manera similar, ¿qué, en tu entorno, produce un sentimiento diferente al sentimiento incómodo que estás experimentando? ¿Qué puedes hacer para provocar este sentimiento?*)
4. Utilizing the following link, identify one of the mindfulness meditations that most appeals to you. There are various themes, lengths, and areas of focus. Which of these helps you feel most soothed? What soothing or calming elements are present for you?

   Link in English: (*Utilizando el siguiente enlace, identifica una de las meditaciones de atención plena que más te atraiga. Hay varios temas, longitudes y áreas de enfoque. ¿Cuál de estos te ayuda a sentirte más aliviado? ¿Qué elementos calmantes o calmantes están presentes para ti? Enlace:*) www.dbtselfhelp.com/html/instant_mindfulness.html
   Link in Spanish: https://ccfwb.uw.edu/resource/meditaciones-guiadas-en-espanol/

 *Quote #2*

"These pains you feel are messengers. Listen to them."
   "Estos dolores que sientes son mensajeros. Escúchalos."

Author: Rumi. He was an Islamic scholar and Maturidi theologian (World, 2019).

**Processing questions for the clients (Preguntas de proceso para los/as clientes)**

1. To what pains do you think Rumi was referring? What pains do you experience most often? (*¿A qué dolores crees que se refería Rumi? ¿Qué dolores experimentas con más frecuencia?*)

2. View the following brief video: Link in English: https://youtu.be/gAMbkJk6gnE. Link in Spanish: www.youtube.com/watch?v=RBOGbgdvfAk

    What does this tell you about the purpose of emotions? (*Ve el siguiente video: https://youtu.be/gAMbkJk6gnE. ¿Qué te dice este sobre el propósito de las emociones?*)

3. If these pains could speak to you, what would they tell you about your life? (*Si estos dolores pudieran hablarte, ¿qué te dirían de tu vida?*)

4. What messages feel most helpful for you at this moment in time? Not all messages, however, should be consumed in their entirety. Which pieces of these messages would you put aside? Why would you leave these pieces behind? (*¿Qué mensajes le resultan más útiles en este momento? Sin embargo, no todos los mensajes deben consumirse en su totalidad. ¿Qué partes de estos mensajes dejarías de lado? ¿Por qué dejarías estas piezas atrás?*)

5. How do you know if these messages are helpful and adaptive or simply believed out of habit? Discuss. (*¿Cómo sabes si estos mensajes son útiles y adaptables o simplemente se creen por costumbre? Discutir.*)

## Quote #3

"Anybody can become angry—that is easy, but to be angry with the right person and to the right degree and at the right time and for the right purpose, and in the right way—that is not within everyone's power and is not easy."

"*Cualquiera puede enojarse, eso es fácil, pero enojarse con la persona adecuada y en el grado correcto y en el momento adecuado y con el propósito correcto, y de la manera correcta, eso no está al alcance de todos y no es fácil.*"

Author: Aristotle. He was a Greek philosopher and polymath during the Classical period in Ancient Greece. Taught by Plato, he was the founder of the Lyceum, the Peripatetic school of philosophy, and the Aristotelian tradition (The Essence of Aristotle's Life, n.d.).

**Processing questions for the clients (Preguntas de proceso para los/as clientes)**

1. Contemplate the quote. Is there a "right" way to experience any of the emotions listed? What role do emotions usually play in your life story? (*Contempla la cita. ¿Existe una forma "correcta" de experimentar alguna de las emociones enumeradas? ¿Qué papel suelen jugar las emociones en la historia de tu vida?*)

2. Consider each emotion that you may be feeling at this moment. These are often layered, so continue exploring beyond the first one or two feelings that you initially identify. Some people may find it helpful to consult a feelings wheel or chart, such as the following: (*Considera cada emoción que puedas estar sintiendo en este momento. A menudo, estas*

*están en capas, así que continúa explorando más allá de los primeros uno o dos sentimientos que identificaste inicialmente. A algunas personas les puede resultar útil consultar una rueda de sentimientos o un gráfico, como el siguiente:)*

Link in English: https://thechalkboardmag.com/the-feelings-circle-chart-emotional-communication

Link in Spanish: http://adriansilisque.com/emociones-basicas-y-una-rueda-de-palabras-emocionales/

3. Imagine each of these emotions as a tool of movement—they either propel you forward, pull you back, pull you down, push you up, or any other direction that comes to mind for you. In what direction does each emotion send you? (*Imagina cada una de estas emociones como una herramienta de movimiento: te impulsan hacia adelante, te empujan hacia atrás, te empujan hacia abajo, te empujan hacia arriba o cualquier otra dirección que se te ocurra. ¿En qué direcciones te envía cada emoción?*)

4. How have these emotions served you in the past? (*¿Cómo te han servido estas emociones en el pasado?*)

5. In what ways might it be helpful to redirect the direction in which these emotions move you? (*¿De qué manera podría ser útil redirigir la dirección en la que te mueven estas emociones?*)

### Quote #4

"Bitterness is like cancer. It eats upon the host. But anger is like fire. It burns it all clean."
   "*La amargura es como el cáncer. Come sobre el anfitrión. Pero la ira es como el fuego. Quema todo limpio.*"

Author: Maya Angelou was an American poet and civil rights activist (2021).

### Processing questions for the clients (Preguntas de proceso para los/as clientes)

1. How do you see the distinctions that are made in this quote? (*¿Cómo ve las distinciones que se hacen en esta cita?*)

2. What is eating at you today? Describe how you are being consumed by the feeling(s)s you are experiencing? (*¿Qué te está comiendo hoy? Describe cómo estás siendo consumido por los sentimientos que estás experimentando.*)

3. In what ways are you a host to your feelings? What parts of you feed these feelings? (*¿De qué manera eres anfitrión de tus sentimientos? ¿Qué partes de ti alimentan estos sentimientos?*)

4. What are the different ways in which the feeling(s) you have identified can show up? What other dimensions or permutations can it take? Which version or permutation will serve to fuel you, rather than harm you? For example, hopelessness can contain elements of grief. Hopelessness can feel all-encompassing and paralyzing, while grief opens a window to honor what has been lost and heal. (*¿Cuáles son las diferentes formas en que pueden manifestarse los sentimientos que has identificado? ¿Qué otras dimensiones o permutaciones*

*pueden tomar? ¿Qué versión o permutación servirá para alimentarte, en lugar de hacerte daño? Por ejemplo, la desesperanza puede contener elementos de duelo. La desesperanza puede ser omnipresente y paralizante, mientras que el dolor abre una ventana para honrar lo que se ha perdido y sanar.)*

5. What might it be like to transform and accept this version of your feeling(s)? Discuss how your story would be different, if you were to adopt this version of your feeling(s). (*¿Cómo sería transformar y aceptar esta versión de sus sentimientos? Discute cómo tu historia sería diferente si adoptaras esta versión de sus sentimientos.*)

## References

Angelou, M. (2021, June 27). www.brainyquote.com/quotes/maya_angelou_148635

Chinese Proverb. (2021, July 1). www.bera.ac.uk/blog/when-the-winds-of-change-blow

*The essence of Aristotle's life.* (n.d.). Mahesh Dutt Sharma.

George, D. (2021, June 7). www.goodreads.com/quotes/72132-may-the-stars-carry-your-sadness-away-may-the-flowers

Hindi Proverb. (2021, January 21). www.daimon.org/lib/proverbs/proverbs-a.htm

Holmes, D. (2021). *Sayings and words of wisdom in English*, p. 50. www.noblepath.info/sayings_and_words_of_wisdom/sayings_and_words_of_wis dom.pdf

World, P. T. (2019). *These pains you feel are messengers to listen to them.* Rumi Journal: 6x9 Inch Dot Grid Bullet Journal/Notebook/Planner/Diary: Inspiring Quote by Rumi—Empowering, Positive, Wisdom, Motivational Poetry, Inspirational Art. (n.p.): Independently Published.

# 13 Courage

In general terms, courage calls for making a decision or taking a series of steps when typically some degree of risk or danger might be involved. This danger might be physical, psychological, or emotional. From a positive standpoint, courage is associated with an internal force that will ensure personal growth. Broadly speaking, most people associate courage with heroic, valiant, or audacious activities such as those performed by police officers, firefighters, military personnel, or individuals who risk their lives in order to save others. Yet, *daily living courage* is the least one talked about as it passes as normal or expected. For instance, it does take courage to raise children and make personal, financial, and physical sacrifices in order to provide for their well-being and support them through all their stages of development. It takes courage for an adolescent to go to school and face microaggressions by bullies on a daily basis. Moreover, it takes courage to keep living while facing a debilitating emotional or physical illness.

It is not difficult to find many types of courage as there are many subcategories that many human beings can relate to when the word courage is mentioned. For instance, *spiritual/existential* courage can be associated with deep meaning questions about life, faith in a higher power, existence, and purpose of living on this earth. Many individuals simply downplay these questions as a denial mechanism and to avoid internal pain. *Affective/emotional courage* is displayed by individuals who are brave enough to confront feelings that have haunted them for years or explore emotions that can potentially open old wounds and endanger current relationships. *Conceptual/intellectual courage* is exhibited when people are willing to explore diverse ideas, principles, and concepts that differ from those learned from their families of origin or culture. For example, the mere exercise of trying to understand the basic tenets of a different political affiliation might be seen as an affront to some but to others is an adventure of analytical courage. *Group/civic/social courage* is demonstrated by individuals who are willing to push the boundaries of normative rules, social expectations, and standard regulations. These individuals risk social embarrassment, isolation, banishment, or total rejection. Even setting a different way of dressing, hair style, and tattoos could be a challenge to the status quo. *Corporeal or tangible courage* is perhaps the most known type of courage in our societies. This is displayed in the form of taking actions at the risk of bodily harm or even potential death. Commonly, it involves some sort of physical resiliency, strength, or endurance. For instance, these would be clearly displayed by individuals who decide to swim for the shore while a ship is adrift in the open sea in order to save the rest of the crew. Or, soldiers who jump on top of a grenade knowing that they will die but in the

DOI: 10.4324/9781003145943-16

process they will save their fellow troopers. Another type of courage is the *honorable, noble, or principled courage* that is manifested in the form of doing the right thing under difficult and compromising situations. This courage is guided by high morals, values, and personal ethics. Ideas are manifested in the form of words and actions that reflect the character of the individual.

See also: humility and self-compassion, patience, self-realization, and focus

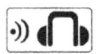 **Microfiction**

### *The Little Kippah*

Paris is not the same as it used to be for us. France has been on high alert since the January 2015 attacks on the Charlie Hebdo offices and a Jewish supermarket in Paris that killed 17 people. Most of my family, including my grandparents, cousins, aunts, and uncles live in a community that is not too far from where these horrific events occurred. Prior to these attacks against the French Jewish population, there had been many antisemitic attacks against Jews on trains and buses. These included physical beatings, throwing glass bottles at us, spitting, and using antisemitic profanity. Many of the members of our Jewish neighborhood who have been here for many generations have left for the United States of America, Spain, and other countries in Latin America. It is the general consensus that safety is paramount and in spite of the government promises, these attacks continue. I am 15 years old and was Bar Mitzvahed two years ago in our local synagogue. It was a moment of tremendous joy as I am now counted as one of the adults in the synagogue and have the privilege to be called to the bimah (platform) to read the Torah (scriptures) in public. I do not understand why people have the capacity to hate others with such intensity. My family are normal people. Papa works as a professor at the university, and mama runs a small newspaper and magazine stand in the block where we live. We are good people, help others as much as we can, and contribute to the community and society at large. Due to the current level of antisemitism and hate, I have been forced to hide my identity. I cannot wear my kippah (skull cap used by Jewish men) in public as I fear for my safety. However, if I keep hiding my identity in a democratic country where all individuals have the right to exercise their freedoms, including the freedom of religion, what does it say about me? Concealing my identity would be tantamount to conceding more power to hate groups. After all, why does a simple piece of cloth in my head (kippah) have to cause so much trouble to others? It is a sign of respect to my Creator and I am not imposing it to anyone else. After consulting with my youth rabbi, he told me that each person has the right to do what is right for them as long as the rights of others are respected. In class, there are some bullies that make fun of me and any time that I want to voice my opinion about my beliefs or my people, they harass me and make fun of me. I am not sure if the teachers are scared of them too or if they share some of their beliefs. I wrote a paper for my history class on antisemitism and its impact in the 20th and 21st centuries.

I mentioned how speech hate evolved into physical abuse and ultimately into political power. Kristallnacht in Germany was the melting point that led into the Holocaust. France, England, Eastern Europe, and the US are facing an unimaginable wave of antisemitism not seen since the times of Hitler. And, it makes me wonder if people forgot in such a short amount of time the devastating effects of one of the greatest genocides committed against humanity. I have made a decision. I will wear my kippah in public while riding the buses or trains. And, I will wear it publicly in class in order to educate others about who we are and why we need to prevent more hate. Instead, all of us need to be part of the solution and not avoid the problem. Evoking the words of "The opposite of love is not hate, but indifference." As a Holocaust survivor and human rights activist, Elie Wiesel dedicated his life to ensuring that humanity would not forget the events under Nazi reign. Of course, I am not Elie Wiesel but my kippah will send a tiny message in the cosmos of hate that can cause ripples of understanding, respect, and courage to respect others!

(*Español*)

 **Microficción**

### *La Pequeña Kipá*

*París no es lo mismo que solía ser para nosotros. Francia había estado en alerta máxima desde los ataques de enero de 2015 contra las oficinas de Charlie Hebdo y un supermercado judío en París que mataron a 17 personas. La mayor parte de mi familia, incluidos mis abuelos, primos, tías y tíos, vive en una comunidad que no está muy lejos de donde ocurrieron estos horribles eventos. Antes de estos ataques contra la población judía francesa, hubo muchos ataques antisemitas contra judíos en trenes y autobuses. Estos incluyen golpes físicos, arrojarnos botellas de vidrio, escupir y usar blasfemias antisemitas. Muchos de los miembros de nuestro barrio judío que han estado aquí durante muchas generaciones se han ido a los Estados Unidos de América, España y otros países de América Latina. El consenso general es que la seguridad es primordial y, a pesar de las promesas del gobierno, estos ataques continúan. Tengo 15 años y fui Bar Mitzvahed hace 2 años en nuestra sinagoga local. Fue un momento de tremenda alegría ya que ahora soy contado como uno de los adultos en la sinagoga y tengo el privilegio de ser llamado a la bimá (plataforma) para leer la Torá (escrituras) en público. No entiendo por qué la gente tiene la capacidad de odiar a los demás con tanta intensidad. Mi familia es gente normal. Papá trabaja como profesor en la universidad y mamá tiene un pequeño quiosco de periódicos y revistas en la cuadra donde vivimos. Somos buenas personas, ayudamos a los demás tanto como podemos y contribuimos a la comunidad y la sociedad en general. Debido al nivel actual de antisemitismo y odio, me he visto obligado a ocultar mi identidad. No puedo usar mi kipá (gorro usado por hombres judíos) en público porque temo por mi seguridad. Sin embargo, si sigo ocultando mi identidad en un país democrático donde todas las personas tienen derecho a ejercer sus libertades, incluida la libertad de religión, ¿qué dice esto de mí? Ocultar mi identidad equivaldría a conceder más poder a los grupos de odio. Después de todo, ¿por qué un simple trozo de tela en mi cabeza (kipá) tiene que causar tantos problemas a los demás? Es una señal de respeto a mi Creador y no se lo estoy imponiendo a nadie más. Después de consultar con el rabino de mi juventud, me dijo que cada persona tiene derecho a hacer lo que sea correcto para él/ella siempre que se respeten los derechos de los demás. En clase, hay algunos bravucones que se burlan de mí y cada vez que quiero expresar mi opinión sobre mis creencias o mi gente, me acosan y se burlan de mí. No estoy seguro de si los profesores también les tienen miedo o si comparten algunas de sus creencias. Escribí un artículo para mi clase de historia sobre el antisemitismo y su impacto en los siglos XX y XXI.*

*Mencioné cómo el discurso de odio se convirtió en abuso físico y finalmente en poder político. Kristallnacht en Alemania fue el punto de fusión que condujo al holocausto. Francia, Inglaterra, Europa del Este y Estados Unidos se enfrentan a una ola inimaginable de antisemitismo no vista desde los tiempos de Hitler. Y me hace preguntarme si la gente olvidó en tan poco tiempo los devastadores efectos de uno de los mayores genocidios cometidos contra la humanidad. He tomado una decisión. Usaré mi kipá en público mientras viajo en autobuses o trenes. Y lo usaré públicamente en clase para educar a otros sobre quiénes somos y por qué debemos prevenir más odio. En cambio, todos debemos ser parte de la solución y no evitar el problema. Evocando las palabras de "Lo opuesto al amor no es el odio, sino la indiferencia". Como sobreviviente del Holocausto y activista de derechos humanos, Elie Wiesel dedicó su vida a garantizar que la humanidad no olvidara los eventos bajo el reinado nazi. Por supuesto, no soy Elie Wiesel, pero mi kipá enviará un pequeño mensaje en el cosmos de odio que puede causar ondas de comprensión, respeto y coraje para respetar a los demás.*

Author: Roberto Swazo.

*Cultural Hints*

The concept of courage can be seen through different cultural prisms. For instance, in Eastern societies courage is seen as a manifestation of millenary values and principles that have been passed down from generation to generation. Many times these are associated with a higher power or intrinsic love for ancestors. In Western culture, courage is manifested by individuals with their particular set of beliefs and personal foundations that at times transcends those of holding average conventional principles.

**Processing questions for the clients (Preguntas de proceso para los/as clientes)**

1. **Empathy question:** Can you put yourself in the shoes of the main character? List the types of feelings that he is experiencing. What feelings resonate more with you? Explain. (***Pregunta de empatía:*** *¿Puedes ponerte en la piel del personaje principal? Enumera los tipos de sentimientos que el personaje está experimentando. ¿Qué sentimientos te resuenan más? Explica.*)

2. Based on the following types of courage, what kind/s of courage is the main character displaying? (a) honorable, noble, or principled courage; (b) corporeal or tangible courage; (c) group/civic/social courage; (d) conceptual/Intellectual courage; (e) affective/emotional courage; and (f) daily living courage. Elaborate. (*Basado en los siguientes tipos de coraje, ¿qué tipo de coraje está mostrando el personaje principal? (a) coraje honorable, noble o basado en principios, (b) coraje corporal o tangible, (c) coraje grupal/cívico/social, (d) coraje conceptual/intelectual, (e) coraje afectivo/emocional, y (f) coraje diario coraje viviente. Elabora.*)

3. Analyze the picture that follows: how do you react when you feel ashamed or put down because of your particular beliefs or ideas? Discuss. (*Analiza la imagen de abajo, ¿cómo reaccionas cuando te sientes avergonzado o desanimado debido a tus creencias o ideas particulares? Discuta.*)

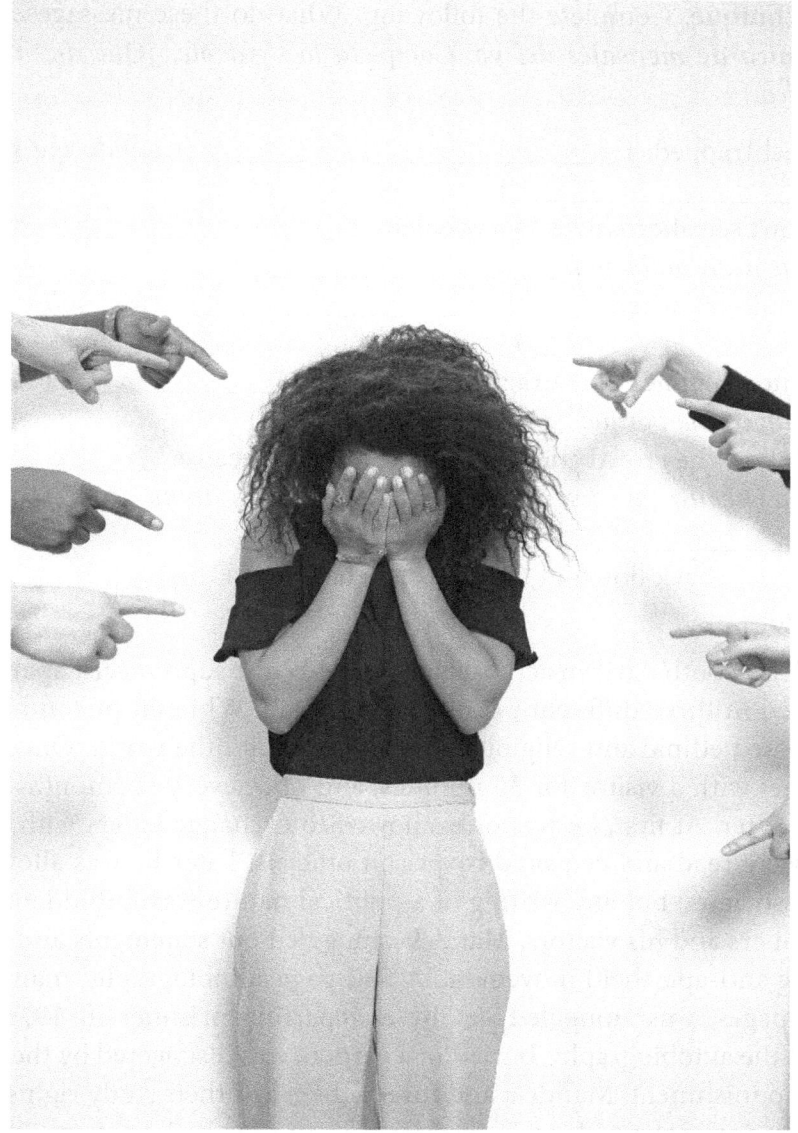

*Figure 13.1* Woman Covering Her Face With Her Hands as Other Hands Point at Her

## Sayings (*dichos*)

### *Saying #1*

"Like a fish, one should look for holes in the net."
   "*Como un pez, uno debe buscar agujeros en la red.*"

Author: Samoan saying (Schultz, 1949).

## Processing questions for the clients (Preguntas de proceso para los/as clientes)

1. What is the main principle taught by this quote? Describe. (*¿Cuál es el principio fundamental que enseña esta cita? Describir.*)

2. **I-message technique**. Complete the following. What do these messages say about you? Explain. (***Técnica de mensajes del yo.*** *Completa lo siguiente. ¿Qué dicen estos mensajes sobre ti? Explica.*)

   a. When I feel trapped, I _____. (*Cuando me siento atrapado,* _____.)

   b. When I don't see alternatives to a problem, I _____. (*Cuando no veo alternativas a un problema,* _____.)

   c. I lack courage when _____. (*Me falta valor cuando* _____.)

   d. I have limited supplies of courage because _____. (*Tengo provisiones limitadas de coraje porque* _____.)

   e. I tend to follow the crowd and rarely make a stand because _____. (*Tiendo a seguir a la multitud y rara vez tomo una posición porque* _____.)

   f. I _____ back down in the face of a challenge. (*Yo* _____ *retrocedo ante un desafío.*)

3. Nelson Mandela (South African activist against the White supremacist apartheid regimen) was imprisoned in three different prisons for 27 years. While in prison he inspired millions of oppressed ethnic and religious minorities around the world. Once a year, he was allowed to meet with a visitor for 30 minutes, and once every six months he could write and receive a letter. At first, he was only allowed to exchange letters with his family, and these letters were read and censored by prison officials. Later he was allowed to write to friends and associates, but any writing of a political nature was forbidden. With the help of fellow prisoners and his visitors, Mandela smuggled out statements and letters to spark the continuing anti-apartheid movement. A 500-page autobiography, manually miniaturized into 50 pages, was smuggled out by a departing prisoner in 1976. The original manuscript of the autobiography, buried in a garden, was discovered by the prison warden soon after. As punishment, Mandela and three others lost their study rights for four years. Being in prison was not an obstacle for Mandela and his beliefs.

***Acting as if technique.*** Act as if you had all the courage and strength of Mandela! How does the new YOU look and act like? Try to explain it and implement it in different ways and areas of your life. Illustrate it.

   [*Nelson Mandela (activista sudafricano contra el régimen de apartheid supremacista blanco) fue encarcelado en tres cárceles diferentes durante 27 años. Mientras estuvo en prisión, inspiró a millones de minorías étnicas y religiosas oprimidas en todo el mundo. Una vez al año, se le permitió reunirse con un visitante durante 30 minutos, y una vez cada seis meses podía escribir y recibir una carta. Al principio, solo se le permitió intercambiar cartas con su familia, y estas cartas fueron leídas y censuradas por los funcionarios de la prisión. Más tarde se le permitió escribir a amigos y asociados, pero se prohibió cualquier escritura de carácter político. Con la ayuda de otros prisioneros y sus visitantes, Mandela sacó de contrabando declaraciones y cartas para impulsar el continuo movimiento contra el apartheid. Una autobiografía de 500 páginas, miniaturizada manualmente en 50 páginas, fue sacada de contrabando por un prisionero que partía en 1976.*

*El manuscrito original de la autobiografía, enterrado en un jardín, fue descubierto por el director de la prisión poco después. Como castigo, Mandela y otras tres personas perdieron sus derechos de estudio durante cuatro años. Estar en prisión no fue un obstáculo para Mandela y sus creencias.*

**La técnica de: actuando como si fuera.** *¡Actúa como si tuvieras todo el coraje y la fuerza de Mandela! ¿Cómo se ve y actúa el nuevo TU? Intenta explicarlo e implementarlo de diferentes formas y áreas de tu vida. Ilustra.)]*

### Saying #2

"If you are afraid of something, you give it power over you."
"*Si le tienes miedo a algo, le das poder sobre ti.*"

Author: Unknown. Moroccan saying (Holmes, 2021, p. 62).

### Processing questions for the clients (Preguntas de proceso para los/as clientes)

1. Many things have power over us and we are unaware of them. We might not be afraid of them per se but we might be afraid of confronting the idea that these do have power over us. Can you identify something or someone that has inspired fear in you throughout your life? Since when have you given him/her/it the power to control aspects of your life? Discuss. (*Muchas cosas tienen poder sobre nosotros y las desconocemos. Puede que no les tengamos miedo en sí, pero podríamos tener miedo de confrontar la idea de que tienen poder sobre nosotros. ¿Puedes identificar algo o alguien que te haya inspirado miedo a lo largo de tu vida? ¿Desde cuándo le has dado el poder de controlar aspectos de tu vida? Discutir.*)

2. Study some biographies of individuals who have conquered their fears and have transformed their lives completely as a result of it. Which one speaks to you the most and why? Explain. (*Estudia algunas biografías de personas que han conquistado sus miedos y han transformado sus vidas por completo como resultado de ello. ¿Cuál te toca más y por qué? Explica.*)

3. Watch this video containing short snippets of information about individuals who conquered their fears with courage and perseverance. Of all of them, which one connects with you the most? That is past failures, pains, disappointments, and disillusionment. Elaborate. (*Mira este video que contiene breves fragmentos de información sobre personas que conquistaron sus miedos con valentía y perseverancia. De todos ellos, ¿con cuál te sientes más conectado? Esto es, fracasos, dolores, decepciones y desilusiones del pasado. Elaborar.*)

www.youtube.com/watch?v=Ydeyl0vXdP0

### Quotes

### Quote #1

"The longest journey begins with the first step."
"*El viaje más largo comienza con el primer paso.*"

Author: Lao-Tzu (Wing-tsit, 2015).

## Processing questions for the clients (Preguntas de proceso para los/as clientes)

1. What is this quote trying to say? Provide several illustrations. (*¿Qué intenta decir esta cita? Proporciona varias ilustraciones.*)

2. A journey is defined differently by many people. A journey can be the beginning of a college degree as a foundation for many other degrees necessary in order to achieve a career very specialized. Or, a journey might be the beginning of a romantic relationship with its ups and downs. Moreover, a journey can be applied to overcoming an addiction or fighting back an illness. Perhaps a journey can be conceptualized for those who have been released from prison and are ready to be reintegrated into a free society.

What is the journey that is or has been in front of you and perhaps has been avoided? Use the image that follows as a mental picture. Remember that a journey is not necessarily traveling physically, but it can be any type of endeavor that requires courage. (*Muchas personas definen un viaje de manera diferente. Un viaje puede ser el comienzo de un título universitario como base para muchos otros títulos necesarios para lograr una carrera muy especializada. O bien, un viaje podría ser el comienzo de una relación romántica con sus altibajos. Además, un viaje se puede aplicar para superar una adicción o combatir una enfermedad. Quizás se pueda conceptualizar un viaje para aquellos que han sido liberados de la prisión y están listos para reintegrarse a una sociedad libre.*

*¿Cuál es el viaje en que estás o ha estado frente a ti y quizás has evitado? Usa la imagen de abajo como una imagen mental. Recuerda que un viaje no es necesariamente un viaje físico, pero puede ser cualquier momento de esfuerzo que requiera coraje.*)

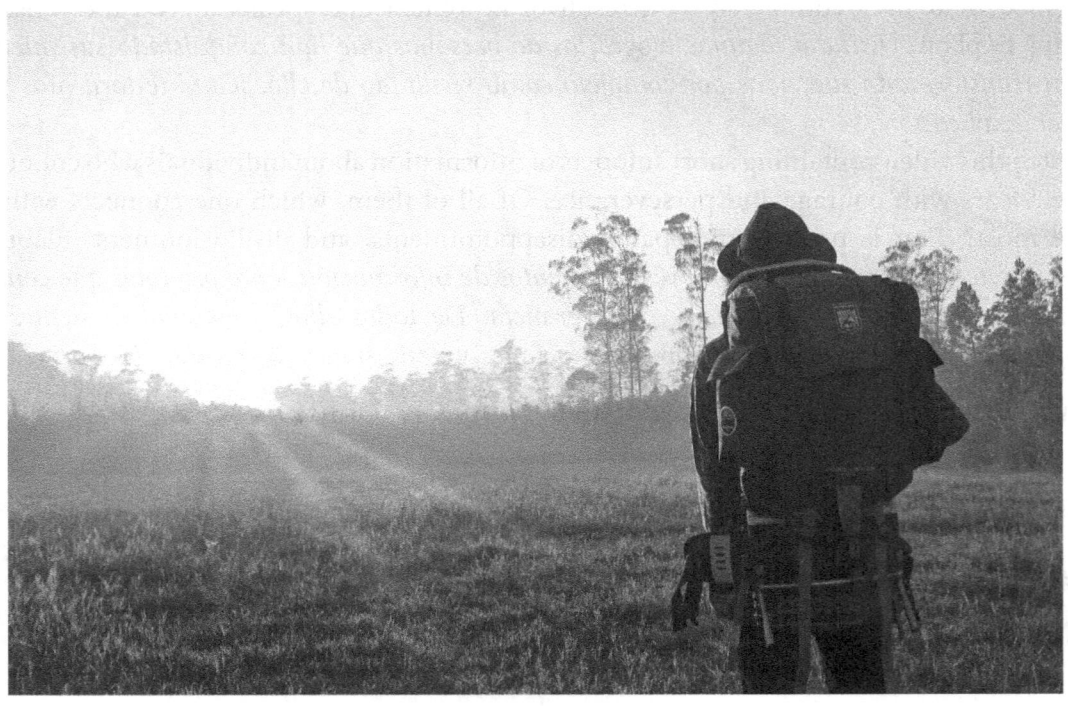

*Figure 13.2* Traveling Person

3. ***Spitting in the soup technique.*** Make a list of all the possible journeys that you have missed in your life because of being afraid of taking a first step. And, go ahead and make a list of all the journeys ahead of you (i.e., physical, social, vocational, financial, spiritual, emotional, relationships). Make a list of all the excuses of not engaging in the very first step. And, because of all these excuses, go ahead and do not embark on any of these journeys. Simply stay where you are at now. Embrace the status quo. Discuss. (***La técnica de escupir en la sopa.*** *Haz una lista de todos los viajes posibles que te has perdido en tu vida por miedo a dar un primer paso. Y haz una lista de todos los viajes que tienes por delante (es decir, relaciones físicas, sociales, vocacionales, financieras, espirituales, emocionales). Haz una lista de todas las excusas para no tomar el primer paso. Y, por todas estas excusas, anímate y no te embarques en ninguno de estos viajes. Simplemente quédate donde estás ahora mismo. Acepta el status quo. Discutir.*)

### Quote #2

"It is easy to be brave from the distance."
   "*Es fácil ser valiente desde la distancia.*"

Author: Aesop (Holmes, 2021, p. 65).

### Processing questions for the clients (Preguntas de proceso para los/as clientes)

1. What does this mean? Examine it and explain. (*¿Qué significa esto? Examínalo y explica.*)
2. ***Paradoxical intention (symptom prescription) technique.*** Go back in time and recall all the times that you have lacked courage and try to put yourself in the same stressful situation/s. In the face of these challenges, behave exactly as you did before, and do it as much as possible. Remain silent and do not advocate for others; stay quiet in the face of racism; laugh when someone engages in microaggressions against multiethnic, racially diverse, and sexual minorities. Keep doing these as much as possible and come back home with your own thoughts. Explain and discuss your internal reactions.

   (***Técnica de intención paradójica (prescripción de síntomas).*** *Retrocede en el tiempo y recuerda todas las veces que te ha faltado coraje y trata de ponerte en las mismas situaciones estresantes. Ante estos desafíos, compórtate exactamente como lo hacía antes y hazlo tanto como sea posible. Permanece en silencio y no defiendas a los demás, quédate callado frente al racismo, ríete cuando alguien se involucre en microagresiones contra minorías multiétnicas, racialmente diversas y sexuales. Sigue haciendo esto tanto como sea posible y vuelve a casa con tus propios pensamientos. Explica y discute tus reacciones internas.*)

3. Distance represents safety but prevents you from doing something for others or yourself due to many reasons such as fear, preventing trouble, etc. Watch the short video clip that follows from John Quinones and explain, what would have you done? Can you cite similar situations in your life and explain how you typically reacted?

   (*La distancia representa seguridad, pero te impide hacer algo por los demás o por ti mismo debido a muchas razones, como el miedo, la prevención de problemas, etc. Mira el breve video de John Quiñones a continuación y explica qué hubieras hecho. ¿Puede citar situaciones similares en tu vida y explica cómo reaccionabas normalmente?)*

www.youtube.com/watch?v=hy2GvPPUGOE

 ### Quote #3

"Be strong and courageous for the Lord is with you wherever you go."
"*Sé fuerte y valiente, porque el Señor estará contigo dondequiera que vayas.*"

Author: Deuteronomy 1 (instructions to Joshua) (King James Bible, n.d.).

 **Processing questions for the clients (Preguntas de proceso para los/as clientes)**

1. Create a mental picture of this dialogue between Moses and Joshua from the Hebrew bible. Moses is the original leader of the Hebrew people who were liberated from the Egyptians and wandered through the desert for 40 years. Joshua is a young, charismatic, passionate, and energetic leader but needs the support of Moses and the assurance that the higher power who delivered their people will be with him.

   How many times have you needed reassurance in your life from someone else who is respected and wise? And, if you have not had this experience before, who do you think can provide this for you in your life? Remember that it does not necessarily have to be a spiritual leader but a person who has a wealth of experience and has accumulated wisdom. Put this in context and start making a list of individuals who can serve as a role model for you. Start having conversations with them individually and establish a person or two that can be your mentors and could instill confidence and courage in your life.

   (*Crea una imagen mental de este diálogo entre Moisés y Josué de la Biblia hebrea. Moisés es el líder original del pueblo hebreo que fue liberado de los egipcios y vagó por el desierto durante 40 años. Josué es un líder joven, carismático, apasionado y enérgico, pero necesita el apoyo de Moisés y la seguridad de que el Poder Superior que liberó a su pueblo estará con él.*

   *¿Cuántas veces has necesitado que alguien más respetado y sabio te tranquilice en tu vida? Y, si no has tenido esta experiencia antes, ¿quién crees que puede proporcionarte esto en tu vida? Recuerda que no necesariamente tienes que ser un líder espiritual sino una persona que tiene una gran experiencia y ha acumulado sabiduría. Pon esto en contexto y comienza a hacer una lista de personas que pueden servirte como modelo a seguir. Empieza a tener conversaciones con ellos individualmente y consolida a una persona o dos que puedan ser sus mentores y puedan infundir confianza y coraje en tu vida.*)

2. **Exploration of spiritual background.** Next is a series of individuals who seek assurance and comfort from a higher power. What are your reactions about these pictures? Explain the positive, negative, and neutral reactions. (***Exploración del trasfondo espiritual.*** *A continuación se muestran una serie de personas que buscan seguridad y consuelo en un poder superior. ¿Cuáles son tus reacciones sobre estas imágenes? Explica las reacciones positivas, negativas y neutrales.*)

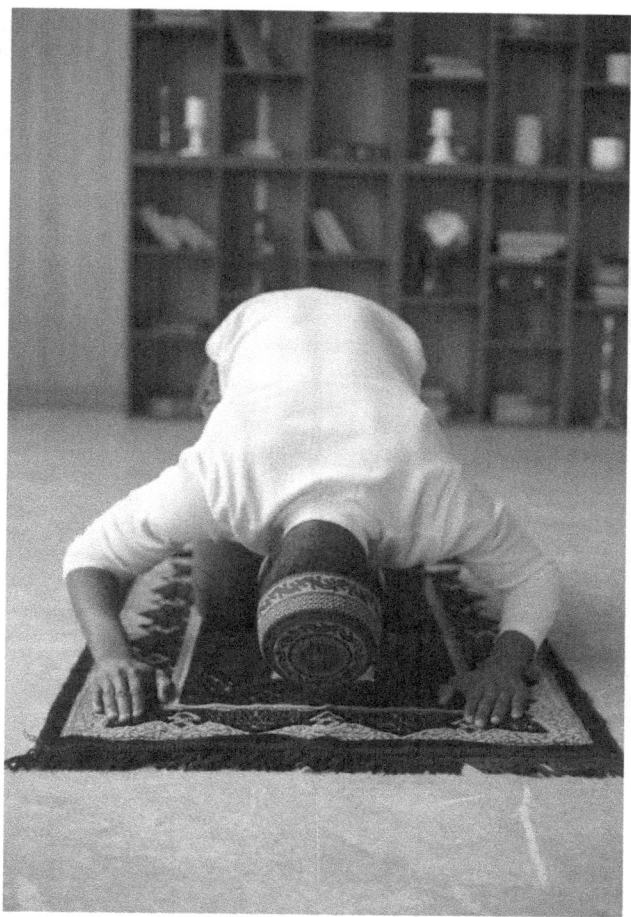

*Figure 13.3*  Muslim Man Praying

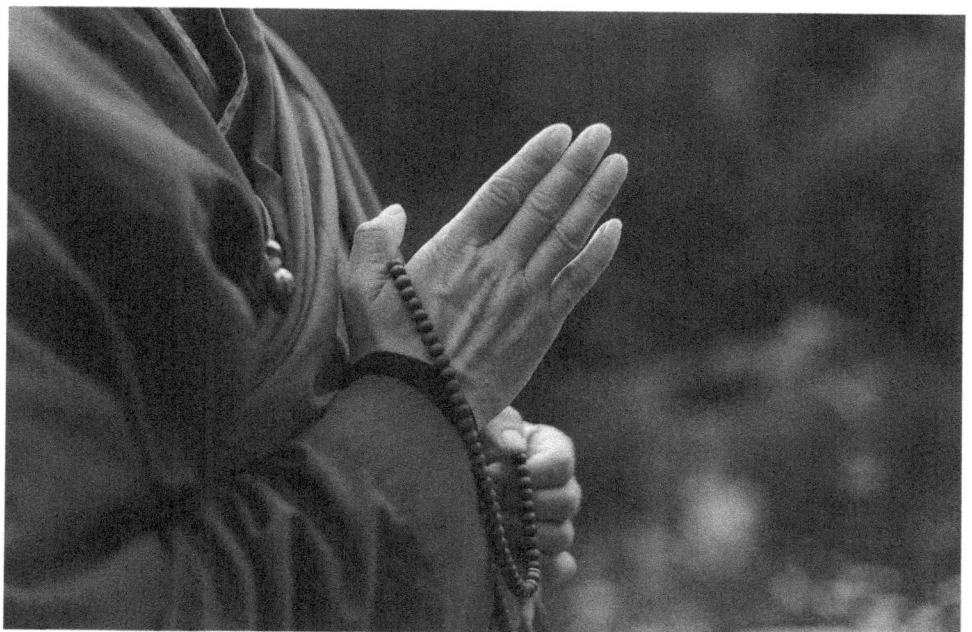

*Figure 13.4*  Hand Holding Prayer Beads

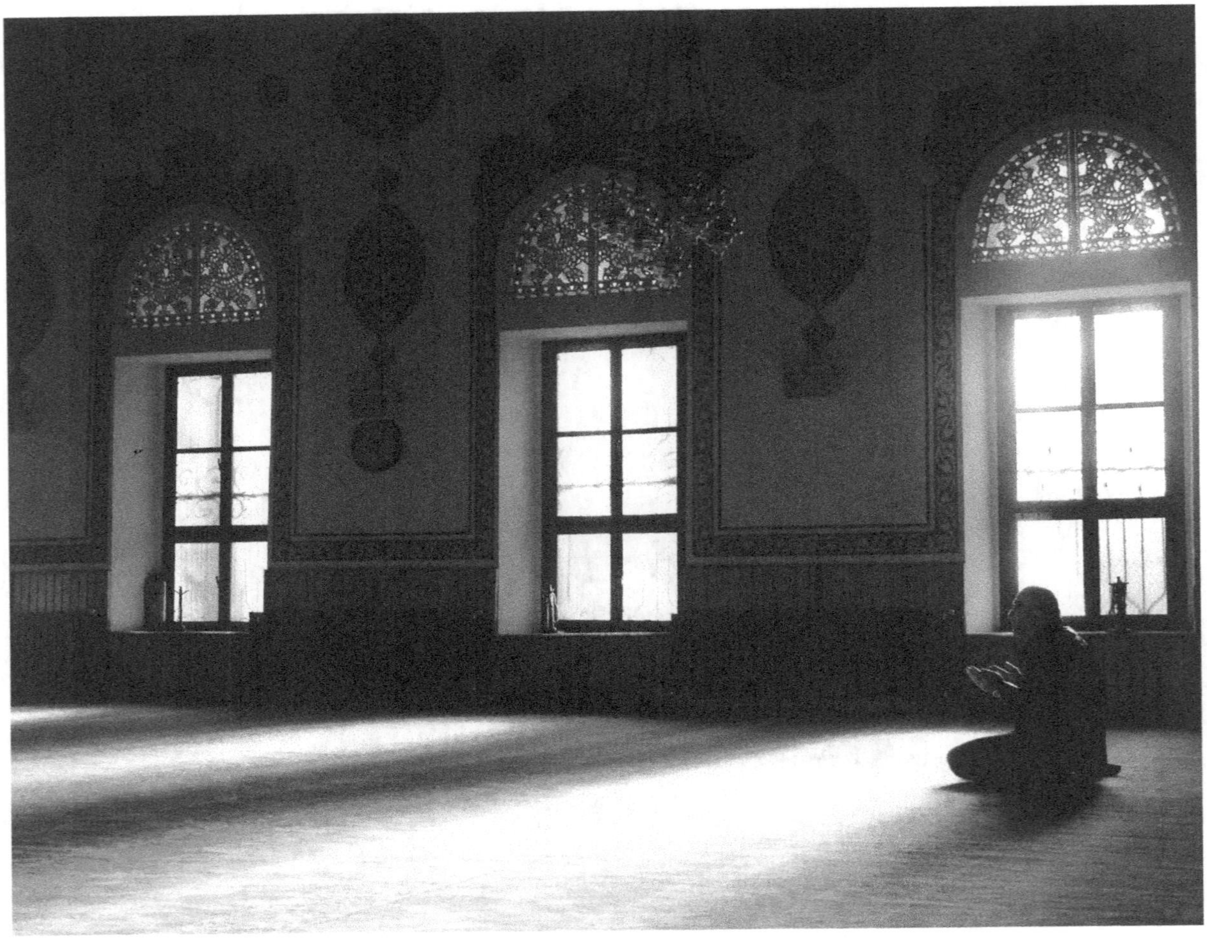

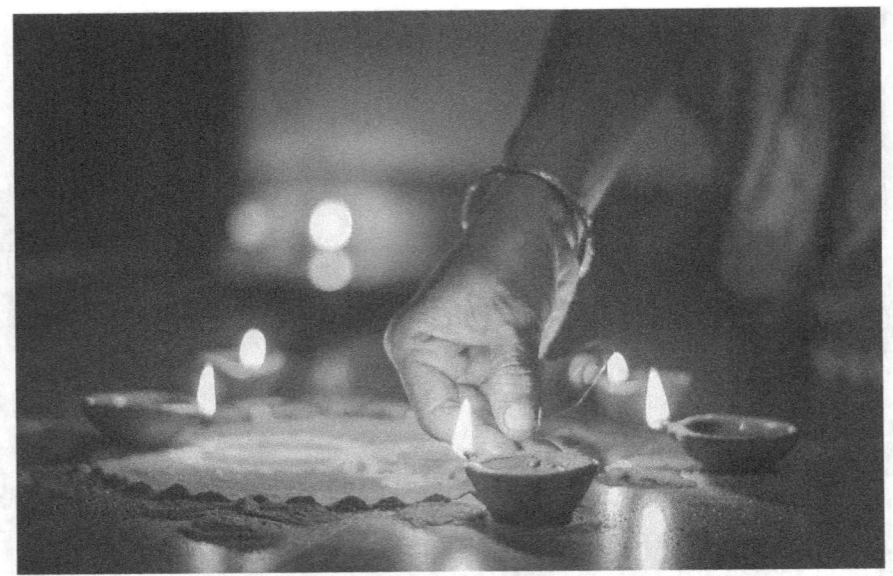

*Figure 13.5*  Man Cross-Legged and Praying With Upturned Hands

*Figure 13.6*  Hand Lighting Religious Candle

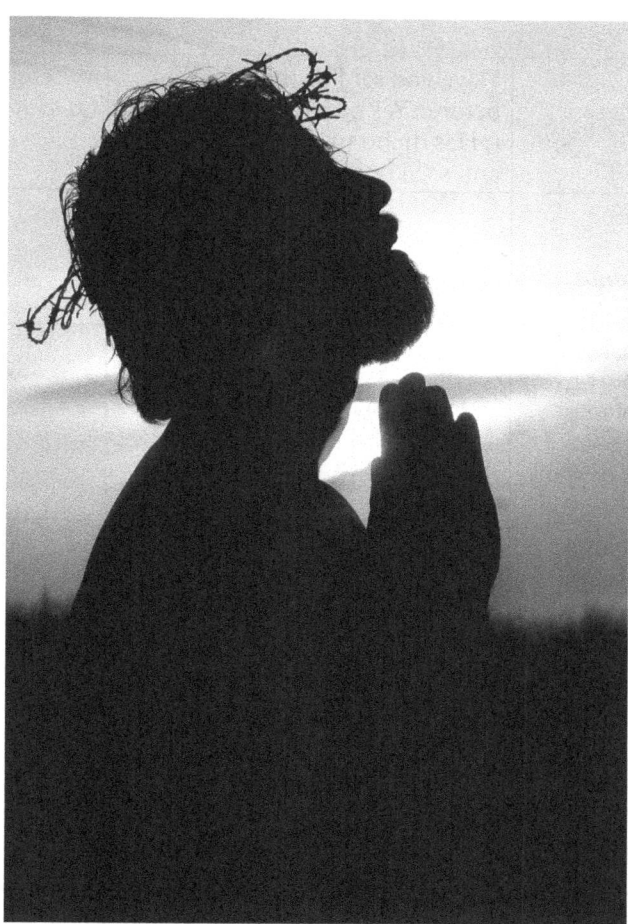

*Figure 13.7* Man Praying

3. Have you ever tried looking for spiritual strength but either negative experiences or lack of knowledge have impeded you from pursuing this? For most human beings, spirituality is not the answer and for others is a journey of exploration. Complete the table that follows and explore your ideas and beliefs. (*¿Alguna vez has intentado buscar la fuerza espiritual, pero las experiencias negativas o la falta de conocimiento te han impedido lograrlo? Para la mayoría de los seres humanos, la espiritualidad no es la respuesta y para otros es un viaje de exploración. Completa la siguiente tabla y explora tus ideas y creencias.*)

*Table 13.1* Exploration of Thoughts and Origins of Spiritual and Religious-Related Thoughts

| Phrase or message (*Frase o mensaje*) | Have you said or thought this before? Yes or No (*¿Has dicho tú o pensado esto antes? Sí o no.*) | Where is this coming from? (*¿De dónde viene esto?*) |
|---|---|---|
| Religion or spirituality is for fanatics (*La religión o espiritualidad es para fanáticos*) | | |

*(Continued)*

*Table 13.1* (Continued)

| Phrase or message (*Frase o mensaje*) | Have you said or thought this before? Yes or No (¿Has dicho tú o pensado esto antes? Sí o no.) | Where is this coming from? (*¿De dónde viene esto?*) |
|---|---|---|
| Most religious people are unintelligent (*La mayoría de las personas religiosas no son inteligentes*) | | |
| Religious people are weak because they need support from something that does not exist (*Las personas religiosas son débiles porque necesitan el apoyo de algo que no existe*) | | |
| Religious people are fanatics (*Las personas religiosas son fanáticas*) | | |
| This world is broken because of religions (*Este mundo está maltrecho por las religiones*) | | |
| Most religions want your money (*La mayoría de las religiones quieren tu dinero*) | | |
| People do crazy things in the name of their religions (*La gente hace locuras en nombre de sus religiones*) | | |
| I don't believe in anything unless I am able to see it, touch it, etc. (*No creo en nada a menos que pueda verlo, tocarlo, etc.*) | | |
| Religious people are hypocrites (*Las personas religiosas son hipócritas*) | | |
| After all, nobody knows what will happen after we die, so what's the big deal (*Después de todo, nadie sabe qué pasará después de nuestra muerte, así que, ¿cuál es el problema?*) | | |
| All that I do and have is because I earn it, I don't owe anything to invisible beings (*Todo lo que hago y tengo es porque me lo gano, no le debo nada a seres invisibles*) | | |

# References

Holmes, D. (2021). *Sayings and words of wisdom in English*, p. 62, p. 65. www.noblepath.info/sayings_and_words_of_wisdom/sayings_and_words_of_wisdom.pdf

King James Bible. (n.d.). *King James Bible Online*. www.kingjamesbibleonline.org/ (Original work published 1769).

Schultz, E. (1949). Proverbial expressions of the Samoans. *Journal of the Polynesian Society*, *58*(4), 139–184. www.jps.auckland.ac.nz/document/?wid=2534

Wing-tsit, C. (2015). *The way of Lao Tzu*. Ravenio Books.

# 14 Patience

During a time when instant gratification is much more feasible, patience seems to be an attribute of the past, a virtue cultivated by mystics who did not have a clue of what productivity, rapid outcomes, and return on investments mean to Western societies. In fact, patience is not a virtue that is frequently taught in schools and promoted by educational standards, in general. Patience does not seem to be a common family value or a pillar of our Western societies. In reality, the opposite is true—the faster one can perform a task, generate an outcome, get an answer, or come up with a product, the more appreciated one will be. We are subjugated by the clicking sounds and beats of our mobile phones, computers, Twitter and Instagram messages, and TikTok accounts. These days, making a line of a couple of people in a bank, supermarket or pharmacy generates anxiety and irritation. Services are expected fast, well done, and without excuses. Speediness is the new normal, anything less than that is simply seen as failure. However, patience in therapy is not only important but necessary. Patience is the fertilizer of reflection and the precursors of internal calmness.

See also: coping, forgiveness, humility and self-compassion, and motivation

 ## Microfiction

### The 2,000-Year-Old Date Seeds

Mama and papa were proud mature and wise date palm trees living in Masada, an ancient site built by the Roman Herod the Great in the 1st century that looked out over the Dead Sea over 2,000 years ago. Papa's name was Methuselah, and mama's name was Edna. They were always attentively looking for their seeds as they wanted to ensure the future of their tree line. During the social and political revolts of different people enslaved and subdued by the Roman Empire, many date trees were lost due to fires. In a desperate attempt to preserve some of their date seeds and future children, Methuselah and Edna talked to some starlings who routinely sought shade under their branches. Methuselah and Edna said to them: "my friends, you have benefitted from our shade and have even built nests for your baby birds on our branches for many years. We only ask of you one favor, we are afraid that our tree line will disappear as a result of human violence and we were wondering if you can secure some date seeds in the most remote corners of the Masada fortress." "Absolutely, Methuselah and Edna, this is the least that we can do for both of you!" the starlings replied. "But do you think that someone will find these beautiful

DOI: 10.4324/9781003145943-17

date seeds some day? Even worse, what if no one finds these date seeds of yours?" "This is a risk that we need to take, my starling friends. Time will tell, time will tell," replied the wise date trees. Two thousand years after the starlings hid the beautiful date seeds in the remote areas of Masada, a couple of Israeli archeologists found some seeds and ran the Carbon 14 test to determine their age. "These are 2,000 years old!" exclaimed the scientists. "What would happen if we planted them?" Taking them back to a similar soil in the area, the scientists planted these seeds and waited, waited, and waited. After almost a full year and at a point in which their hopes were almost gone, a series of small plants started to sprout! Then, eight years later, people were eating plump dates that were literally over 2,000 years old. Methuselah and Edna were right: "time will tell, time will tell."

Author: Roberto Swazo.

*Note:* This story was inspired by the seeds found in Israel that were found in Masada (Israel) and dated to be over 2,000 years old.

 *Cultural Hints*

Patience is not seen as a modern value in our Western society, but it is a typical value in most Eastern societies. Therefore, you might have to tailor and edit the questions based on your population in order to increase the levels of relevance.

(*Español*)

 **Microficción**

### Las Semillas de Dátiles de 2,000 Años

*Mamá y papá eran unas orgullosas palmeras de dátiles maduras y sabias que vivían en Masada, un antiguo sitio construido por el romano Herodes el Grande en el siglo I que miraba hacia el Mar Muerto hace más de unos 2,000 años atrás. El nombre de papá era Matusalén y el de mamá era Edna. Siempre estaban protegiendo atentamente sus semillas, ya que querían asegurar el futuro de su línea ancestral. Durante las revueltas sociales y políticas de diferentes pueblos esclavizados y sometidos por el Imperio Romano, muchos árboles de dátiles se perdieron debido a los incendios. En un intento desesperado por preservar algunas de sus semillas de dátiles y sus futuros hijos, Matusalén y Edna hablaron con algunos estorninos que rutinariamente buscaban sombra bajo sus ramas. Matusalén y Edna les dijeron: "Amigos míos, ustedes se han beneficiado de nuestra sombra e incluso han construido nidos para sus pajaritos en nuestras ramas durante muchos años. Solo les pedimos un favor, tememos que nuestra línea de árboles desaparezca como resultado de la violencia humana y nos preguntábamos si pueden esconder nuestras semillas de dátiles en los rincones más recónditos de la fortaleza de Masada. "¡Absolutamente Matusalén y Edna, esto es lo mínimo que podemos hacer por ustedes dos! ¿Pero creen que alguien encontrará estas hermosas semillas de dátiles algún día? Peor aún, ¿qué pasa si nadie encuentra estas semillas de dátiles? Este es un riesgo que tenemos que llevar mis amigos estorninos. El tiempo lo dirá, el tiempo lo dirá ". Respondieron los sabios árboles de dátiles. Dos mil años después de que los estorninos escondieron las hermosas semillas de dátiles en las áreas remotas de Masada, un par de arqueólogos israelíes encontraron algunas semillas y realizaron la prueba de carbono 14 para determinar su edad. "¡Estas tienen 2000 años!" "Exclamaron los científicos". "¿Qué pasaría si las sembramos? Lleván- dolos de regreso a un suelo similar en el área, los científicos sembraron estas semillas y esperaron, esperaron y esperaron. Después de casi un año y en un punto en el que sus esperanzas casi se habían acabado, ¡una serie de pequeñas plantas comenzaron a brotar! Luego, 8 años después, la gente estaba comiendo dátiles deliciosos que tenían literalmente más de 2,000 años. Matusalén y Edna tenían razón: "el tiempo lo dirá, el tiempo lo dirá."*

**Processing questions for the clients (Preguntas de proceso para los/as clientes)**

1.  What is your initial reaction after reading the story? (*¿Cuál es tu reacción inicial después de leer la historia?*)
2.  Describe your opinion about Methuselah and Edna? What are your thoughts about their plan? Explain. (*Describe tu opinión sobre Matusalén y Edna. ¿Cuáles son tus pensamientos sobre su plan? Explicar.*)
3.  They had to wait 2,000 years for the outcome of their plan to materialize, and yet, they did not actually see the outcome, but it happened. Do you think that you would have that kind of patience and faith for an outcome? Provide some illustrations. (*Tuvieron que esperar 2,000 años para que se materializara el resultado de su plan y, sin embargo, en realidad no vieron el resultado, pero sucedió. ¿Crees que tendrías ese tipo de paciencia y fe para obtener un resultado? Proporciona algunas ilustraciones.*)
4.  Why was patience so important to them? And, if you could go back in time, when would you have exercised patience of this type in the past? Any regrets? Discuss. (*¿Por qué era tan importante para ellos la paciencia? Y, si pudieras retroceder en el tiempo, ¿cuándo habrías ejercido una paciencia de este tipo en el pasado? ¿Te arrepientes? Discutir.*)

**Sayings (*dichos*)**

*Saying #1*

"When you were a hammer you had no mercy, now that you are an anvil, be patient."
    *"Cuando fuiste martillo no tuviste clemencia, ahora que eres yunque, ten paciencia."*

Author: Unknown. Popular Spanish saying (R. Vallestejo, personal communication, June 7, 2017).

**Processing questions for the clients (Preguntas de proceso para los/as clientes)**

1.  What is the meaning of this saying? (*¿Cuál es el significado de este dicho?*)
2.  At what times of your life have you been a hammer? And, when have you been an anvil? Provide specific illustrations. The picture that follows may help you stimulate your thought process. (*¿En qué momentos de tu vida has sido un martillo? Y, ¿cuándo has sido un yunque? Proporciona ilustraciones específicas. La siguiente imagen puede ayudarte a estimular tu proceso de pensamiento.*)

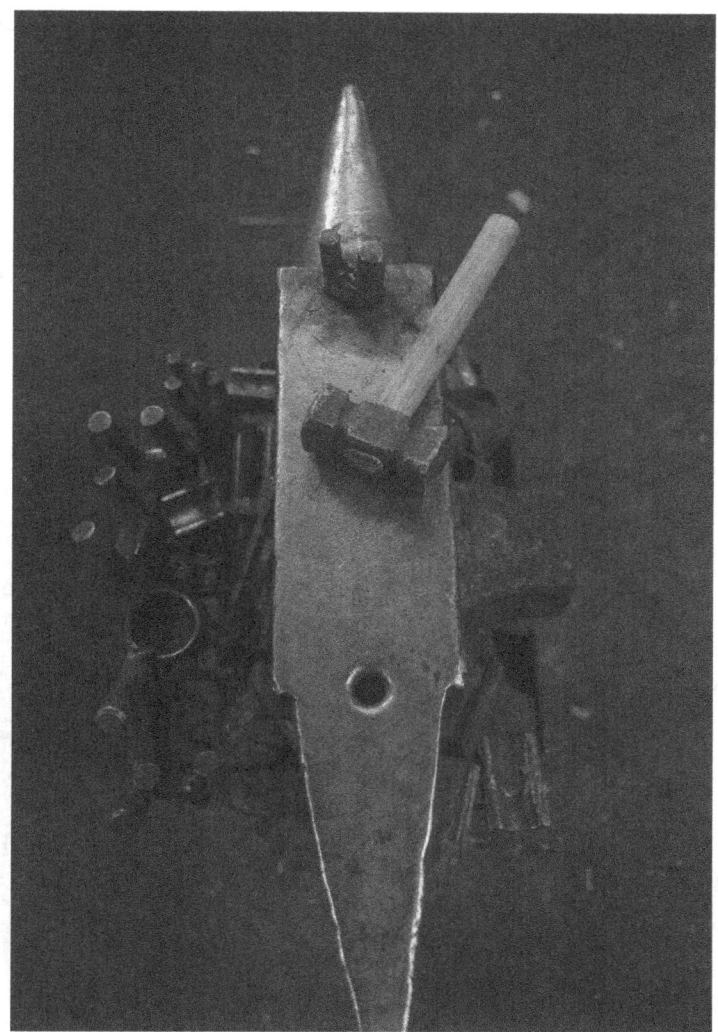

*Figure 14.1* Hammer and Anvil

3. How did you handle being an anvil, and who did you blame for being in that position? Explain. (*¿Cómo manejaste el ser un yunque y a quién culpaste por estar en esa posición? Explicar.*)
4. Did you apply the gained knowledge and evolve? Or, were you angry during the entire process? (*¿Aplicaste los conocimientos adquiridos y evolucionaste? ¿O estuviste enojado/a durante todo el proceso?*)

 *Saying #2*

> "Patience is a tree with bitter roots but very sweet fruits."
> "*La paciencia es un árbol de raíz amarga pero de frutos muy dulces.*"

Author: Unknown. Persian saying (GameLEN, 2021).

**Processing questions for the clients (Preguntas de proceso para los/as clientes)**

1. Describe the image of a tree that follows. What is the representation of the sweet fruits in your life? Elaborate. (*Describe el árbol de abajo. ¿Cuál es la representación de los frutos dulces en tu vida? Elaborar.*)

2. What is the meaning of the bitter roots in your life? Describe. (*¿Cuál es el significado de las raíces amargas en tu vida? Describir.*)

3. Knowing that the soil makes a substantial difference in the life and development of a tree, what kinds of soil (conditions, sites, people, locations, etc.) have helped you to develop patience or have impeded you to grow in patience? Discuss. (*Sabiendo que el suelo hace una diferencia sustancial en la vida y el desarrollo de un árbol, ¿qué tipo de suelo (condiciones, sitios, personas, lugares, etc.) te han ayudado a desarrollar la paciencia o te han impedido crecer en paciencia? Discutir.*)

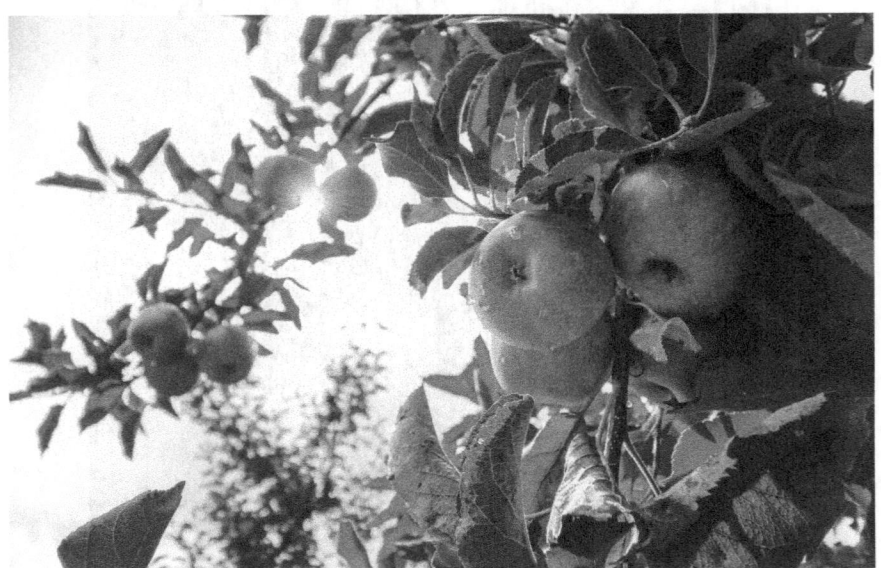

*Figure 14.2* Fruitful Apple Tree

## Quotes

 *Quote #1*

"Patience is simply more than learning to wait. It is having learned what is worth your time."
   "*La paciencia es simplemente más que aprender a esperar. Es haber aprendido lo que vale tu tiempo.*"

Author: Jonathan Muncy Storm is an American writer (2021). He has no formal academic background and is a mechanic by training who decided to start writing in his spare time.

 *Cultural Hints*

Time and patience are interconnected and feed off each other. Working with traditional North American clients can take some time to nurture these concepts as they are not intrinsically attached to the culture. Patience is not necessarily a virtue that is complimented in Western culture, instead speediness, promptness, and quick reactions are associated with productivity. Patience is associated with growth and inner growth in Eastern cultures.

 **Processing questions for the clients (Preguntas de proceso para los/as clientes)**

1. Break down the quote in two parts and provide examples that are connected to your daily activities. (*Divide la cita en dos partes y proporciona ejemplos relacionados con sus actividades diarias.*)

2. Based on the picture that follows, what can you say about this person? Look at the mannerism, how many times have you behaved like this? (*Basado en la imagen de abajo, ¿qué dice eso sobre esta persona? Mira el manerismo, ¿cuántas veces te has comportado así?*)

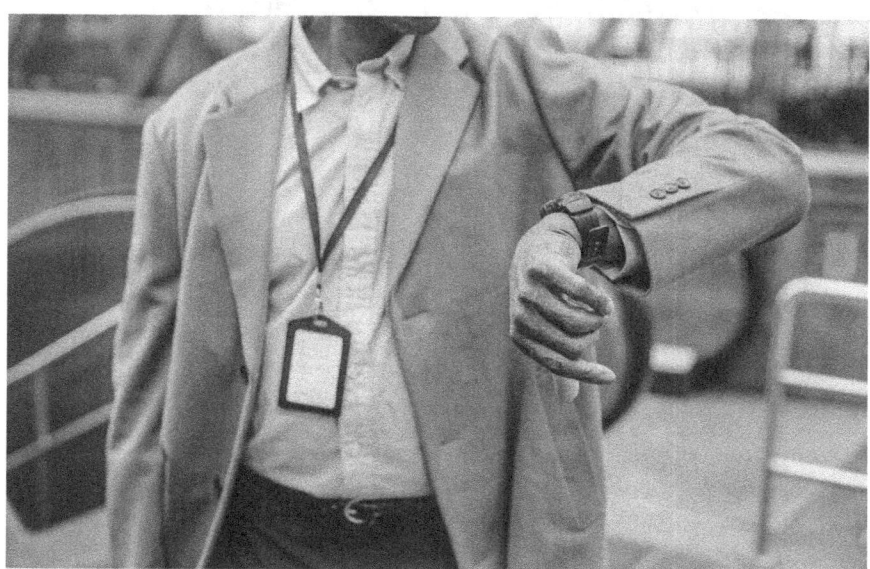

*Figure 14.3* Man Looking at His Watch

3. What is worth waiting patiently for in your life? And, what is not? List and discuss. (*¿Qué vale la pena esperar pacientemente en tu vida? ¿Y qué no lo es? Enumera y discute.*)

 *Quote #2*

"Patience is a form of wisdom. It demonstrates that we understand and accept the fact that sometimes things must unfold in their own time."

*"La paciencia es una forma de sabiduría. Demuestra que comprendemos y aceptamos el hecho de que a veces las cosas deben desarrollarse en su propio tiempo."*

Author: Dr. Joh Kabat-Zinn. Scientist, writer, and meditation teacher who has applied mindfulness principles to traditional medicine (2013).

 **Processing questions for the clients (Preguntas de proceso para los/as clientes)**

1. See the picture that follows; imagine that you are the last person driving a car within the sea of vehicles. You are scheduled to be at an important meeting in 1 hour and you

realize that you will not be able to escape this traffic jam for over 2 hours. (*Ve la imagen a continuación; imagina que eres la última persona que conduce un automóvil dentro del mar de vehículos. Estás programado para estar en una reunión importante en 1 hora y te das cuenta de que no podrás escapar de este atasco durante más de 2 horas.*)

2. Close your eyes and imagine the intensity of the traffic. What kind of thoughts are going through your mind? Have you ever been in a similar situation? Explain. (*Cierra los ojos e imagina la intensidad del tráfico. ¿Qué tipo de pensamientos pasan por tu mente? ¿Has estado alguna vez en una situación similar? Explicar.*)

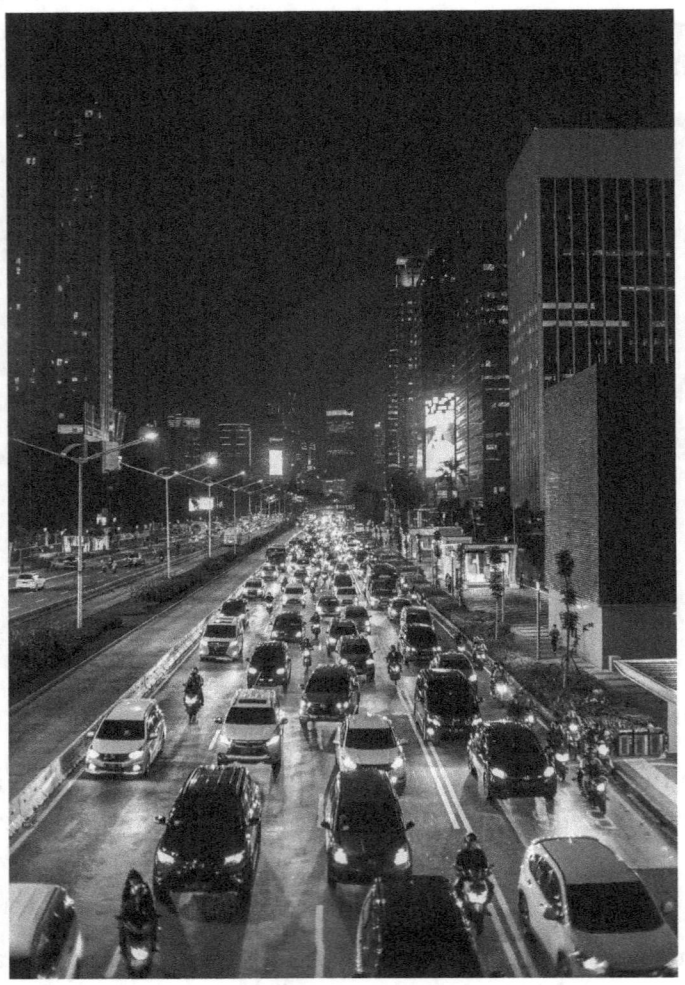

*Figure 14.4*  Traffic Jam at Night

3. Do you typically accept that things must unfold in their own time? If not, how do you handle this? Analyze. (*¿Aceptas normalmente que las cosas deben desarrollarse a su debido tiempo? Si no es así, ¿cómo manejas esto? Analizar.*)

4. Provide a series of illustrations of times in which things needed to go through their own process and were not able to unfold in spite of your anxiety. Example: finishing high school, college, pregnancy, etc. (*Proporciona una serie de ilustraciones de momentos en los que las cosas debían pasar por su propio proceso y no pudieron desarrollarse a pesar de tu ansiedad. Ejemplo: terminar la escuela secundaria, la universidad, el embarazo, etc.*)

***Quote #3***

> "With love and patience nothing is impossible."
> *"Con amor y paciencia nada es imposible."*

Author: Daisako Ikeda, Japanese Buddhist philosopher, educator, author, and nuclear disarmament advocate (2021).

 *Cultural Hints*

In this era of extreme individualism, love seems to be devoted only to those close to us and even in a conditional way. Love for others is typically delegated to individuals with deep religious convictions who are seeking collective well-being and harmony. This is a very foreign concept for many individuals living in toxically divided and polarized societies in which winning and taking advantage of others is more important than caring for them.

**Processing questions for the clients (Preguntas de proceso para los/as clientes)**

1. From the table that follows, circle the emotions that you experience when you experience a lack of patience. And, on the opposite side, indicate what precise event or situation triggered it and how you handled it. (*En la siguiente tabla, marca con un círculo las emociones que sientes cuando experimentas falta de paciencia. Y, en el lado opuesto, indica qué evento o situación precisa lo desencadenó y cómo lo manejaste.*)

*Table 14.1* Emotional Triggers or Activators and Ways of Handling Each

| Emotions (*Emociones*) | Trigger and how it was handled (*Detonador y como se manejo*) |
|---|---|
| • Admiration (*admiración*)<br>• Adoration (*adoración*)<br>• Aesthetic Appreciation (*Apreciación estética*)<br>• Amusement (*diversión*)<br>• Anxiety (*ansiedad*)<br>• Awkwardness (*torpeza*)<br>• Boredom (*aburrimiento*)<br>• Calmness (*calma*)<br>• Confusion (*confusión*)<br>• Craving (*antojo*)<br>• Disgust (*asco*)<br>• Empathetic pain (*dolor empático*)<br>• Envy (*envidia*)<br>• Excitement (*emoción*)<br>• Fear (*miedo*)<br>• Horror (*horror*)<br>• Interest (*interes*)<br>• Joy (*alegría*)<br>• Nostalgia (*nostalgia*)<br>• Romance (*romance*)<br>• Sadness (*tristeza*)<br>• Satisfaction (*satisfacción*)<br>• Sexual desire (*deseo sexual*)<br>• Sympathy (*simpatía*)<br>• Triumph (*triunfo*) | |
| | Additional comments:<br><br>(*comentarios adicionales*) |

2. Love is a highly complex emotion that has many layers and can be expressed and directed toward different people, animals, symbols, organizations, and higher beings. Are you able to associate the virtue of patience with any of these? How is it expressed? Explain. (*El amor es una emoción muy compleja que tiene muchas capas y puede expresarse y dirigirse hacia diferentes personas, animales, símbolos, organizaciones y seres superiores. ¿Puedes asociar la virtud de la paciencia con alguno de estos? ¿Cómo se expresa? Explicar.*)

3. Creating your own Patience Long-Term Plan. (*Creación de tu propio plan de paciencia a largo plazo.*)

   a. Patience is associated with better mental health. Is the lack of patience robbing you from quality mental health? How often do you experience depressive and anxiety symptoms? How do you cope with these? (*La paciencia está asociada con una mejor salud mental. ¿La falta de paciencia te está robando de una calidad de salud mental? ¿Con qué frecuencia experimentas síntomas de depresión y ansiedad? ¿Cómo los manejas?*)

   b. **Build new friendships** within your neighborhood, social and religious circles, and at work. Is patience an issue as you try to establish these relationships? Elaborate. (**Construye nuevas amistades** *dentro de tu vecindario, círculos sociales y religiosos y en el trabajo. ¿Es la paciencia un problema al intentar establecer estas relaciones? Elaborar.*)

   c. **Rethink your goals.** Make a list and determine how many of these require patience and how you are currently coping with these. (**Reconsidera tus metas.** *Haz una lista y determina cuántos de estos requieren paciencia y cómo los estás enfrentando actualmente.*)

   d. **Physical health.** The lack of patience is associated with the following: headaches, acne flare-ups, ulcers, diarrhea, insomnia, irritability, muscle pain, and pneumonia among others. Visit your physician and get a full check up to see what are the current health gaps that you are experiencing. Identify if any of these are linked to a lack of patience and the emotions attached to it. (**Salud física.** *La falta de paciencia se asocia con lo siguiente: como dolores de cabeza, brotes de acné, úlceras, diarrea, insomnio, irritabilidad, dolores musculares y neumonía entre otros. Visita a tu médico y hazte un chequeo completo para ver cuáles son las brechas de salud actuales que estás experimentando. Identifica si alguna de estas está relacionada con la falta de paciencia y las emociones asociadas a ella.*)

## References

GameLEN. (2021, August 27). *The wisdom of the proverb.* https://gamelen.com/en/the-wisdom-of-the-proverb/

Ikeda, D. (2021, March 22). www.goodreads.com/quotes/68777-with-love-and-patience-nothing-is-impossible

Kabat-Zinn, J., & Hanh, T. N. (2013). *Full catastrophe living: Using the wisdom of your body and mind to face stress, pain, and illness* (Revised ed.). Random House Publishing Group.

Storm, J. M. (2021, October 26). www.passiton.com/inspirational-quotes/8077-patience-is-more-than-simply-learning-to-wait#:~:text=%E2%80%9CPatience%20is%20more%20than%20simply,%E2%80%94J.M.%20Storm%20%7C%20PassItOn.com

# Part III

# Mindfulness

## Reflection and Wellness

# 15 Focus

Focus is defined as to concentrate on something in particular. Focus can be conceptualized as to bring into view. An example of focus is to put all of one's energy into a writing, science, or music project. According to the Merriam-Webster Dictionary (n.d.), focus is

> defined as a center of activity, attraction, or attention, a point of concentration, directed attention, emphasis, direction, a state or condition permitting clear perception or understanding, adjustment for distinct vision or the area that may be seen distinctly or resolved into a clear image.

In the counseling profession, and according to the International Focusing Institute:

> the name 'Focusing' is not used in the conventional idea of focused attention. Rather, Gene Gendlin chose this word as a metaphor for the process of recognizing vague, subtle, or ephemeral somatic sensations that could gradually be brought into focus, as one might adjust a pair of binoculars to turn a blurry visual image into clear, recognizable objects. We usually capitalize the word 'Focusing' in order to indicate that we mean it in this particular way. Once a felt sense has come into focus (meaning it is more present, clear, and stable) one can move to the step Gendlin calls 'asking.' Simple questions like 'What are you worried about?' or 'What do you need?' are addressed to the felt sense itself, as if talking with a friend. Often (not always) if one waits patiently and gently, the felt sense will answer with an unexpected insight, an 'Aha!' moment, along with a body sense of release or opening (often referred to as a 'shift'). Something held deep inside has come unstuck, providing a new sense of direction and fresh energy to undertake it.

In an era of inattentiveness and distractibility due to scattered interests in which technology, politics, sports, and fantasy narratives dominate the landscape, our clients have difficult times reorienting themselves into a personal centeredness. Since most clients are unaware of their own scattered inner worlds and how these are reflected on their own lives, the challenge of the counselor is to help the client to find methods to live more meaningful lives.

See also: goals, future, inspiration, patience, and self-realization

DOI: 10.4324/9781003145943-19

## Microfiction

### *The Legend of the Squirrels and Monkeys*

The father told his children to turn off the television, leave behind any type of electronic devices, and maybe bring with them one book, notebook, and a pencil. Disgruntled, the children protested and started asking questions about this decision. The father told them that they were going to spend a full day in the forest.

"An entire day without TV, playing electronic games or checking our tablets? That is impossible, dad. Are you trying to punish us? We have not done anything wrong!" The father stared at his little children with a compassionate look and told them: "I will show you a secret that very few know about but the only way that I can teach you this secret is by going to the forest in person." The idea of a secret, and most particularly going to the forest, sparked some interest in the children. The children and the father packed some fresh fruits, nuts, dried fish, bread, cheese, and vegetables into their bags for the forest adventure. After arriving at the edge of the forest, the father parked the car, and each of the children carried their backpacks with them, including the book, notebook, and pencil. It was beautiful in the middle of the spring. They walked for a couple of hours with short breaks for water and a snack. Strategically, the father found a place that was full of leafy trees with lots of different animals and birds nesting around. He put a big blanket on the ground and told the children to take a short nap to freshen up. After the nap, the father told them to read the book that they brought with them for one hour without interruptions. Curiously, the children followed the instructions with very little resistance. After an hour of reading, the father served them lunch, and told them to take notes or draw what they saw on the trees. They drew pictures of energetic squirrels and little spider monkeys jumping around from one branch to the next. After a while the father asked the children if they knew about the legend of the origin of monkeys and squirrels. Immediately, and with a sense of curiosity they said that they did not know about this legend. The father proceeded to ask them, "What do you notice about squirrels and monkeys?" They immediately said that they are jumping, moving, twitching, scratching, fighting, and chasing each other most of the time. Then, the father asked them if they knew why? They did not know why, and asked him what was going on? The father told them that there is a legend that says that monkeys and squirrels used to be people, human beings. Right away, the children were intrigued by this initial introduction. Their eyes opened up very wide and told him that it was impossible!

"Okay, okay. Let me tell you and you be the judge, alright? The legend says that there was a big group of people who entered a magic forest in which all wishes could be granted. The magic forest was full of all kinds of things that one could possibly imagine. They simply needed to formulate a thought and whatever it was it could come true. Anything is possible. Suddenly, these people were thinking about many possibilities and things were coming to fruition. They thought about food, money, jewels, clothing, houses, and all kinds of things. They also started to try to outdo each other by getting more things. Since their thoughts were coming to reality, the disorganization of their thoughts became more and more disruptive and out of control. Their own thoughts got in the way of their own physical reactions and they started looking around, scratching, flexing, twitching, running, jumping, and chasing each other. With time, their bodies started to change more and more to the point that they lost total control of their own thoughts. Since they could not think straight, they lost complete focus of their reality and their own identities. They became total mental chaos. The years passed and they became monkeys and squirrels."

The father said: "Do you understand why these squirrels and monkeys around us are jumping around, scratching, twitching, and doing things with no clear purpose? These are the descendants of the original people who went to the magic forest." The children were in disbelief and mesmerized at the chaotic behavior of the monkeys and squirrels. The father declared: "You are who you are because either you control or don't control your thoughts. If you cannot focus on one thing, then, it is very likely that your reality is reactive to multiple things that most likely are not important." At the end of the day, the children had read more from the book and had conversed with the father for an extended period of time. Their walk toward the car was mostly contemplative while looking with pity at the monkeys and squirrels who were clowning around.

*(Español)*

 ### Microficción

### *La Leyenda de las Ardillas y los Monos*

*El padre les dijo a sus hijos que apagaran la televisión, dejaran cualquier tipo de dispositivo electrónico y tal vez trajeran un libro, una libreta y un lápiz. Los niños, descontentos, protestaron y empezaron a hacer preguntas sobre esta decisión. El padre les dijo que iban a pasar un día completo en el bosque.*

*"¿Un día entero sin televisión, jugando juegos electrónicos o revisando nuestras tabletas? Eso es imposible papá. ¿Estás tratando de castigarnos? ¡No hemos hecho nada malo! "El padre miró a sus pequeños con una mirada compasiva y les dijo: "Les mostraré un secreto que muy pocos conocen, pero la única forma en que puedo enseñarles este secreto es yendo al bosque en persona". La idea de un secreto y, sobre todo, de ir al bosque, despertó cierto interés en los niños. Los niños y el padre empacaron algunas frutas frescas, nueces, pescado seco, pan, queso y verduras en sus bolsas para la aventura por el bosque. Después de llegar al borde del bosque, el padre estacionó el auto y cada uno de los niños llevó consigo sus mochilas, incluido el libro, la libreta y el lápiz. Era hermoso en medio de la primavera. Caminaron durante un par de horas con breves descansos para tomar agua y un refrigerio. Estratégicamente, el padre encontró un lugar lleno de árboles frondosos con muchos animales y pájaros diferentes anidando alrededor. Puso una gran manta en el suelo y les dijo a los niños que tomaran una pequeña siesta para refrescarse. Después de la siesta, el padre les dijo que leyeran el libro que habían traído durante una hora sin interrupciones. Curiosamente, los niños siguieron las instrucciones con muy poca resistencia. Después de una hora de lectura, el padre les sirvió el almuerzo y les dijo que tomaran notas o dibujaran lo que veían en los árboles. Hicieron dibujos de ardillas enérgicas y pequeños monos araña saltando de una rama a la siguiente. Después de un rato, el padre preguntó a los niños si conocían la leyenda del origen de los monos y las ardillas. De inmediato, y con cierto sentido de curiosidad, dijeron que no conocían esta leyenda. El padre procedió a preguntarles, "¿qué notan sobre las ardillas y los monos?" Inmediatamente dijeron que saltaban, se movían, se retorcían, se rascaban, peleaban y se perseguían la mayor parte del tiempo. Entonces, el padre les preguntó si sabían por qué. No sabían por qué y le preguntaron qué estaba pasando. El padre les dijo que hay una leyenda que*

*dice que los monos y las ardillas solían ser personas, seres humanos. De inmediato, los niños se sintieron intrigados por esta presentación inicial. ¡Sus ojos se abrieron mucho y le dijeron que era imposible!*

*"Bien bien. Déjame decirte y tú serás el juez, ¿de acuerdo? La leyenda dice que hubo un gran grupo de personas que se adentraron en un bosque mágico en el que se podían conceder todos los deseos. El bosque mágico estaba lleno de todo tipo de cosas que uno podría imaginar. Simplemente necesitaban formular un pensamiento y, fuera lo que fuera, podía hacerse realidad. Cualquier cosa es cualquier cosa. De repente, estas personas estaban pensando en muchas cosas y las cosas se estaban convirtiendo en realidad. Pensaron en comida, dinero, joyas, ropa, casas y todo tipo de cosas. También empezaron a intentar superarse entre sí consiguiendo más cosas. Dado que sus pensamientos se estaban volviendo realidad, la desorganización de sus pensamientos se volvió cada vez más perturbadora y fuera de control. Sus propios pensamientos se interpusieron en el camino de sus propias reacciones físicas y comenzaron a mirar a su alrededor, rascarse, flexionarse, retorcerse, correr, saltar y perseguirse unos a otros. Con el tiempo, sus cuerpos comenzaron a cambiar cada vez más hasta el punto de perder el control total de sus propios pensamientos. Como no podían pensar con claridad, perdieron el enfoque completo de su realidad y sus propias identidades. Se convirtieron en un caos mental total. Pasaron los años y se convirtieron en monos y ardillas."*

*El padre dijo: "¿Entiendes por qué estas ardillas y monos que nos rodean están saltando, rascando, retorciéndose y haciendo cosas sin un propósito claro? Estos son los descendientes de las personas originales que fueron al bosque mágico". Los niños estaban incrédulos y hipnotizados por el comportamiento caótico de los monos y las ardillas. El padre declaró: "Eres quien eres porque o controlas o no controlas tus pensamientos. Si no puede concentrarse en una cosa, entonces, es muy probable que su realidad reaccione a varias cosas que probablemente no sean importantes." Al final del día, los niños habían leído más del libro y habían conversado con el padre durante un largo período de tiempo. Su caminata hacia el auto fue mayormente contemplativa mientras miraban con lástima a los monos y ardillas que hacían payasadas.*

Author: Roberto Swazo.

·)) 🎧  **Processing questions for the clients (Preguntas de proceso para los/as clientes)**

1. What is the essence of this story? What called your attention the most? Explain. (*¿Cuál es la esencia de esta historia? ¿Qué te llamó más la atención? Explica.*)

2. How much control do you have over your thought process? How can you prevent behaving like a squirrel or a monkey? Discuss. (*¿Cuánto control tienes sobre tu proceso de pensamiento? ¿Cómo evitar comportarse como una ardilla o un mono? Discutir.*)

3. Mindfulness and focusing exercise: (*Ejercicio de atención plena y concentración:*)

   a. Close your eyes and imagine one task or something that you want to achieve or obtain. This can be a physical object or an activity. (*Cierra los ojos e imagina una tarea o algo que quieras lograr u obtener. Puede ser un objeto físico o una actividad.*)

   b. Picture it vividly in your mind and eliminate all types of distractions. (*Imagínelo vívidamente en su mente y elimine todo tipo de distracciones.*)

   c. Focus completely on it as if there was nothing else in the world. (*Concéntrese completamente en él como si no hubiera nada más en el mundo.*)

d. Determine how much time you need to accomplish this. Calculate this into your daily activities. (*Determina cuánto tiempo necesitas para lograrlo. Calcule esto en sus actividades diarias.*)

e. If you are getting off track, again, close your eyes briefly, take a deep breath, and refocus again. (*Si se está desviando, de nuevo, cierre los ojos brevemente, respire hondo y vuelva a concentrarse.*)

f. Refocusing is about being in the moment and controlling your state of mind and eventual actions. (*Reenfocarse se trata de estar en el momento y controlar su estado mental y acciones eventuales.*)

g. Repeat this process based on your daily activities and evaluate your outcomes at the end of the week. Repeat on a daily basis. (*Repita este proceso según sus actividades diarias y evalúe sus resultados al final de la semana. Repite a diario.*)

 **Sayings (*dichos*)**

 *Saying #1*

"The wolf does not need someone to bring him food, his survival instinct focuses him on getting it."

"*El lobo no necesita que alguien le traiga la comida, el instinto de supervivencia lo enfoca a conseguirla.*"

Author: Jewish Sephardi saying (G. Azoulay, personal communication, March 17, 2020).

**Processing questions for the clients (Preguntas de proceso para los/as clientes)**

1. There is something instinctual about focusing on something that does not need to be taught or reinforced. The basic needs of seeking shelter, food, water, air, safety, sleep, and clothing are instilled in our human DNA of survival. Obviously, wolves have basic instincts like human beings. What can you learn about the intense focus for survival of the wolves and how it differs from yours as a human being? Explain. (*Hay algo instintivo en concentrarse en algo que no necesita ser enseñado o reforzado. Las necesidades básicas de buscar refugio, comida, agua, aire, seguridad, sueño y ropa están inculcadas en nuestro ADN humano de supervivencia. Obviamente, los lobos tienen instintos básicos como los seres humanos. ¿Qué puedes aprender sobre el intenso enfoque para la supervivencia de los lobos y en qué se diferencia del tuyo como ser humano? Explicar.*)

2. Let's assume that you have satisfied all your basic needs as stated in the previous question, what is preventing you from focusing on obtaining the things that you want in life? Elaborate. (*Supongamos que ha satisfecho todas sus necesidades básicas como se indicó en la pregunta anterior, ¿qué le impide concentrarse en obtener las cosas que desea en la vida? Elaborar.*)

3. The opposite of focusing is being distracted. A distraction is a way to avoid a situation and not confront it head on. Make a list of all the distractions that are preventing you from focusing on yourself, a task, or a goal. Be specific. (*Lo opuesto a enfocar es distraerse. Una distracción es una forma de evitar una situación y enfrentarla de frente. Haz una lista de todas las distracciones que te impiden concentrarte en ti mismo, una tarea o una meta. Se específico.*)

**Quotes**

 *Quote #1*

"It's very important that we re-learn the art of resting and relaxing. Not only does it help prevent the onset of many illnesses that develop through chronic tension and worrying; it allows us to clear our minds, focus, and find creative solutions to problems."

*"Es muy importante que volvamos a aprender el arte de descansar y relajarse. No solo ayuda a prevenir la aparición de muchas enfermedades que se desarrollan a través de la tensión crónica y la preocupación; nos permite aclarar nuestras mentes, concentrarnos y encontrar soluciones creativas a los problemas."*

Author: Thích Nhất Hạnh. He is a Vietnamese Thiền Buddhist monk, peace activist, and founder of the Plum Village Tradition (Schnall, 2017).

**Processing questions for the clients (Preguntas de proceso para los/as clientes)**

1. The author defines resting and relaxing as an art. What does he mean by it? Explain. (*El autor define descansar y relajarse como un arte. ¿Qué quiere decir con eso? Explicar.*)
2. **Detox plan for relaxation improvement**: The following table will help you track your weekly activities and determine if there is an unbalance between work and relaxation. (*Plan de Desintoxicación para Mejorar la Relajación: la siguiente tabla lo ayudará a realizar un seguimiento de sus actividades semanales y determinar si existe un desequilibrio entre el trabajo y la relajación.*)

*Table 15.1* Plan for Relaxation Improvement Activity

| Day of the week (*Dia de la semana*) | Number of working hours (*Número de horas de trabajo*) | Relaxation activities (*Actividades de relajación*) | Hours of sleep (*Horas de sueño*) | Number of hours in front of a screen (i.e., phone, TV, computer) (*Número de horas frente a una pantalla (es decir, teléfono, TV, computadora)*) | Improvement plan (*Plan de mejora*) |
|---|---|---|---|---|---|
| Monday (*lunes*) | | | | | |
| Tuesday (*martes*) | | | | | |
| Wednesday (*miércoles*) | | | | | |
| Thursday (*jueves*) | | | | | |
| Friday (*viernes*) | | | | | |
| Saturday (*sábado*) | | | | | |
| Sunday (*domingo*) | | | | | |
| | Total (*total*) | Summary (*resumen*) | Total (*total*) | Total (*total*) | |

3. When was the last time you took an entire weekend off without any working activities? And, when was the last time that you booked a week or more of real vacation time without checking your phone or email for work related activities? What does it say about you, your priorities, and lifestyle? Explain. (*¿Cuándo fue la última vez que se tomó un fin de semana libre sin ninguna actividad laboral? Y, ¿cuándo fue la última vez que reservó una semana o más de vacaciones reales sin consultar su teléfono o correo electrónico para ver las actividades relacionadas con el trabajo? ¿Qué dice sobre ti, tus prioridades y tu estilo de vida? Explicar.*)

 **Quote #2**

"Censorship no longer works by hiding information from you; censorship works by flooding you with immense amounts of misinformation, of irrelevant information, of funny cat videos, until you're just unable to focus."

"*La censura ya no funciona ocultándote información; la censura funciona inundándote con inmensas cantidades de desinformación, de información irrelevante, de videos graciosos de gatos, hasta que no puedes concentrarte.*"

Author: Yuval Noah Harari. He is an Israeli public intellectual, historian, and a professor in the Department of History at the Hebrew University of Jerusalem (2017).

 **Processing questions for the clients (Preguntas de proceso para los/as clientes)**

1. Describe your initial reaction to the content of this quote. What comes to your mind as you read it? Unpack your answer as much as you can. (*Describe tu reacción inicial al contenido de esta cita. ¿Qué te viene a la mente mientras lo lees? Desempaquete su respuesta tanto como pueda.*)

2. Are you able to fully describe the difference between being fully concentrated into something and the times when you were not? Clarify. (*¿Eres capaz de describir completamente la diferencia entre estar completamente concentrado en algo y los momentos en los que no lo estabas? Aclarar.*)

3. Acquiring centeredness is not an automatic process by any means; reshifting your focus requires establishing routines, breaking down old patterns, and taking control of your thought process, emotions, and environment. It is probably easier to follow the distractions around you and get lost on the Internet rather than complete a task or invest time in your own cognitive processes. Reaching self-focus is intimately connected to self-control. And, if you are not in self-control, something or somebody has some inherent control over your life. By not being focused you are feeling frustrated and dissatisfied with yourself and those around you. Take a day off by yourself. Do not bring your children, significant others, relatives, or friends. Do not turn on the radio, watch TV, or browse the Internet. Read, meditate, eat well, and concentrate on your own thought process. Identify what is dominating your thoughts and what are the predominant themes and emotions associated with them. Journal your thoughts throughout the day. Repeat this in a week or two. Start identifying patterns that are leading you to be unfocused and scattered. How can these be overcome? Demonstrate. (*Adquirir la centralidad no es un proceso automático de ninguna manera, cambiar su enfoque requiere establecer rutinas, romper viejos patrones y tomar el control de su proceso de pensamiento, emociones y entorno. Probablemente sea*

*más fácil seguir las distracciones que te rodean y perderte en Internet en lugar de completar una tarea o invertir tiempo en tus propios procesos cognitivos. Alcanzar el enfoque en uno mismo está íntimamente relacionado con el autocontrol. Y, si no tienes autocontrol, algo o alguien tiene algún control inherente sobre tu vida. Al no estar concentrado, te sientes frustrado e insatisfecho contigo mismo y con los que te rodean. Tómate un día libre. No traiga a sus hijos, seres queridos, parientes o amigos. No encienda la radio, no mire televisión ni navegue por Internet. Lea, medite, coma bien y concéntrese en su propio proceso de pensamiento. Identifique qué está dominando sus pensamientos y cuáles son los temas y emociones predominantes asociados con ellos. Escribe tus pensamientos a lo largo del día. Repita esto en una semana o dos. Empiece a identificar patrones que lo lleven a estar desenfocado y disperso. ¿Cómo se pueden superar? Demostrar.)*

 **Quote #3**

"The key to success is to focus our conscious mind on things we desire, not things we fear."
    *"La clave del éxito es enfocar nuestra mente consciente en las cosas que deseamos, no en las cosas a las que tememos."*

Author: Brian Tracy. He is a Canadian-American motivational public speaker and self-development author (2014).

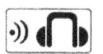 **Processing questions for the clients (Preguntas de proceso para los/as clientes)**

1. Based on this quote, are you able to identify the things that you desire and things that you fear? Most importantly, which ones tend to be the predominant ones in your life? And, how much time do you devote to them, both the ones that you fear and the ones that you desire? Elaborate. (*Con base en esta cita, ¿eres capaz de identificar las cosas que temes y temes? Más importante aún, ¿cuáles tienden a ser las predominantes en tu vida? Y, ¿cuánto tiempo les dedicas, tanto a los que temes como a los que deseas? Elaborar.*)

2. Photograph exercise. In order to increase your focus, complete the following exercise: (*Ejercicio de fotografía. Para aumentar su concentración, complete el siguiente ejercicio:*)

    a. Take a picture or photograph of something that you desire. This can be a specific material object such as a house, car, location, object, etc. Or, this can be something more abstract such as love, peace, spiritual growth, or wealth in general, and the picture or photograph exemplifies the meaning of this. (*Toma una foto o fotografía de algo que desees. Puede ser un objeto material específico, como una casa, un automóvil, un lugar, un objeto, etc. O puede ser algo más abstracto, como el amor, la paz, el crecimiento espiritual o la riqueza en general, y la imagen o fotografía ejemplifica el significado de esta.*)

    b. Dedicate four specific times during the day to the following exercise. (*Dedica 4 momentos específicos del día al siguiente ejercicio.*)

    c. In the morning, immediately when you wake up and before looking at your phone, news, or any negative source of information, take this photograph and stare at it for 5 minutes straight. Keep ALL your focus into it. Avoid any distractions from people, sounds, or external sources. Repeat this at noon, late afternoon, and before going to bed. (*Por la mañana, inmediatamente cuando te despiertes y antes de mirar tu teléfono, noticias o cualquier fuente de información negativa, toma esta fotografía y mírala durante 5 minutos seguidos. Mantenga TODO su enfoque en ello. Evita cualquier distracción de personas, sonidos o fuentes externas. Repita esto al mediodía, al final de la tarde y antes de acostarse.*)

d.  Immediately after staring and focusing on the photograph for 5 minutes, close your eyes, and keep this mental image in your mind. Do not let anything or anyone disturb this image. (*Inmediatamente después de mirar fijamente y enfocar la fotografía durante 5 minutos, cierre los ojos y mantenga esta imagen mental en su mente. No dejes que nada ni nadie perturbe esta imagen.*)

e.  Most importantly, think about this photograph as if it were real in your life. The important part is to increase the focus and transport the image from your mind into your life. Remember, focus on what you want and not the excuses or the obstacles for not getting it! (*Lo más importante es que piense en esta fotografía como si fuera real en su vida. La parte importante es incrementar el enfoque y transportar la imagen de tu mente a tu vida. Recuerda, céntrate en lo que quieres y no en las excusas o los obstáculos para no conseguirlo.*)

3.  Focusing music exercise. (*Ejercicio de música de enfoque.*)

a.  Find a quiet place at home before starting any activity. Have a list of all the things that you want to accomplish during the day. Read them several times, prioritize based on order of importance. (*Busque un lugar tranquilo en casa antes de comenzar cualquier actividad. Tenga una lista de todas las cosas que quiere lograr durante el día. Léalos varias veces, priorice según el orden de importancia.*)

b.  Play the following YouTube music: (*Reproduce la siguiente música de YouTube:*) www.youtube.com/watch?v=sjkrrmBnpGE

c.  Visualize each of the items on your list done at the end of the day. (*Visualice cada uno de los elementos de su lista hechos al final del día.*)

d.  Focus solely on the items and ignore any kind of distractions. (*Concéntrese únicamente en los elementos e ignore cualquier tipo de distracción.*)

e.  Take a deep breath, hold it, slowly exhale, and repeat for a few minutes. (*Respire profundamente, retenga la respiración, exhale lentamente y repita durante unos minutos.*)

f.  Remember that your imagination is the most powerful tool, and this subconscious mind will become a reality if you prevent any unwanted distractions from polluting your mental space. (*Recuerda que tu imaginación es la herramienta más poderosa y esta mente subconsciente se convertirá en una realidad si evitas distracciones no deseadas que contaminen tu espacio mental.*)

## Quote #4

"By putting a date on a dream, it becomes a goal. A goal divided into steps becomes a plan. And a plan supported by actions becomes a reality."

*"Al ponerle fecha a un sueño se convierte en meta. Una meta dividida en pasos se convierte en un plan. Y un plan apoyado por acciones se vuelve realidad."*

Author: Greg Reid (Reid, 2021).

 **Processing questions for the clients (Preguntas de proceso para los/as clientes)**

1. How can you best describe the meaning of this quote? (*¿Cómo puede describir mejor el significado de esta cita? Describir.*)
2. In order to evolve from a dream into a goal, and break it down into steps toward a plan that is converted into action, one must have something internal or external helping to get to the final point. If you are lacking it, how does this force look to you? Explain. (*Para evolucionar de un sueño a una meta, y dividirlo en pasos hacia un plan que se convierte en acción, uno debe tener algo interno o externo que ayude a llegar al punto final. Si te falta, ¿cómo te parece esta fuerza? Explicar.*)
3. Using the analogy of lenses, how can you create the ideal "prescribed lenses" for your current situation? How do they need to be adjusted? Elaborate. (*Utilizando la analogía de los lentes, ¿cómo puede crear los "lentes recetados" ideales para su situación actual? ¿Cómo deben ajustarse? Elaborar.*)

## References

Harari, Y. N. (2017). *Homo deus: A brief history of tomorrow.* Harper.

Merriam-Webster. (n.d.). Focus. In *Merriam-webster.com dictionary.* Retrieved June 18, 2021, from https://www.merriam-webster.com/dictionary/focus

Reid, G. (2021, May 9). *Quotes.* www.goodreads.com/quotes/7119798-a-dream-written-down-with-a-date-be Comes-a-goal

Schnall, M. (2017, December 6). Exclusive interview with zen master Thích Nhất Hạnh. *Huffington Post.* www.huffpost.com/entry/beliefs-buddhism-exclusiv_b_577541

Tracy, B. [@BrianTracy]. (2014, December 16). The key to success is to focus our conscious mind on things we desire, not things we fear [Tweet]. *Twitter.* https://twitter.com/BrianTracy/status/548478853879197696

# 16 Goals

Goals is perhaps one of the most used terms in counseling and therapy in general. When clients come to us for services or when they are referred by other professionals, the key idea is to accomplish a series of goals that demonstrate change and growth. It is very rare to enter into a counseling relationship without having determined goals that will lead the entire process. Unlike other species, human beings have the ability to conceptualize the future and visualize a specific outcome based on current actions. While most species base their existence on obtaining shelter, food, and procreation, human beings are able to operate in an abstract dimension that allows them to produce an outcome that is not immediate. For instance, we might engage in a long-term goal by getting married, having children, purchasing a home, starting a small business, losing weight, preparing for years to qualify for the Olympics, grow spiritually, and gain political experience to become a mayor or senator. Similarly, we can develop life learning goals in which aside from formal degrees, learning becomes a lifestyle. Similarly we can pursue personal development goals in order to be a better person overall and achieve happiness in the process. Or perhaps, we can pursue relationship goals with the idea of repairing family relationships or romantic partnerships. Within the aforementioned, these can be framed between short-term and long-term goals. In essence, goals are abstract ideas that are operationalized with day-to-day activities converting them into tangible expressions of the inner thoughts, feelings, and desires of an individual. As therapists, helping clients to achieve their goals is one of the most important and gratifying aspects of our profession.

See also: future, focus, inspiration, patience, and motivation

 **Microfiction**

### The Box With 24 Gold Ingots

Walking on an isolated road, a man rested under the shade of a large tree. There were many rocks under the tree and the man found a soft spot among the rocks with the purpose of evading the hot hours of the day before continuing his journey. While resting, a flat rock with freshly removed ground around it called his attention. He lifted it up and noticed a wooden box with 24 gold ingots. Immediately, he looked around to see if this was some type of trap or joke. He waited and waited but no one was near this isolated area. The note read: "If you found this note, it means that the 24 gold ingots are yours. Keep in mind that every morning at 12:01 am, a new set of 24 gold ingots will be placed in here. If you do not pick them up at the end of 24 hours,

DOI: 10.4324/9781003145943-20

that is, 11:59 pm, these will be removed and you cannot claim them. Another set of 24 gold ingots will be placed but the previous ones cannot be claimed and therefore are lost. You cannot send anyone to pick these up, from now on, only you can do it." Of course, the man thought that this was a tasteless joke and his skeptical personality obligated him to walk to the closest town to test the value of the 24 gold ingots. It took him almost a full walking day in order to get to the closest town. To his surprise, they were real! Now, he needed to go back to the rocky side under the tree to see if the box had been replenished with gold ingots. After resting a full day in town, he was restless because he knew that if the note was true, a set of gold was already lost by 11:59 pm. The next day, he bought a camel and traveled to the site in half a day. The box had another set of 24 gold ingots! Immediately, these were packed in his bag. After a few hours of rest, he took off again with his tired camel. Since the camel had not rested enough and replenished itself with water, it collapsed and died half way. He kept walking frantically to town to test the goal again. Yes! These are real! Now, he needed to put these somewhere and come back for more. The man decided to purchase a big semi-abandoned farm in order to bury the golden ingots in an isolated spot close to the barn. He bought a caravan of camels, supplies, water jugs, dry food, and protective gear against the intense heat with the purpose of protecting the camels. Once he arrived in the deserted area, he camped with the intention of staying for a month and collecting the highest amount of gold possible. He collected a total of 720 gold ingots and was ready to head back to the farm. Once on the farm, he buried these along with the others. He rested a day, and immediately repeated the process. He bought fresh camels and traveled to the deserted area to collect more gold ingots. He spent the last years of his life repeating traveling, collecting gold ingots, going back to the farm, burying them, and heading back for more. In spite of the fact that he was immensely wealthy, he never bought anything other than supplies and camels for the multiple journeys. He never invested the gold, bought properties, donated to those in need, or simply exchanged part of it in currency in order to get a return on his investment. All the gold was simply buried underground, nothing came out of it.

(*Español*)

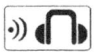 ## Microficción

### *La Caja con los Lingotes de 24 Kilates*

*Caminando por un camino aislado, un hombre descansaba bajo la sombra de un gran árbol. Había muchas rocas debajo del árbol y el hombre encontró un lugar blando entre las rocas con el propósito de pasar las horas calurosas del día antes de continuar su viaje. Mientras descansaba, una roca plana con tierra recién removida a su alrededor llamó su atención. La levantó y vio una caja de madera con 24 lingotes de oro. Inmediatamente, miró a su alrededor para ver si se trataba de algún tipo de trampa o broma. Esperó y esperó, pero no había nadie cerca de esta área aislada. La nota decía: "Si encontró esta nota, significa que los 24 lingotes de oro son suyos. Tenga en cuenta que todas las mañanas a las 12:01 am, se colocará aquí un nuevo juego de 24 lingotes de oro. Si no las recoge al cabo de 24 horas, es decir, a las 11:59 pm, estas se retirarán y no podrá reclamarlas. Se colocará otro juego de 24 lingotes de oro pero los anteriores no se pueden reclamar y por lo tanto se pierden. No puede enviar a nadie a recogerlos, de ahora en adelante, sólo usted puede hacerlo". Por supuesto, el hombre pensó que se trataba de una broma de mal gusto y su personalidad escéptica lo obligó a caminar hasta el pueblo más cercano para probar el valor de los 24 lingotes de oro. Le tomó casi un día completo de caminata para llegar al pueblo más cercano. Para su sorpresa, ¡eran reales! Ahora, necesitaba volver al lado rocoso debajo del árbol para ver si la caja estaba llena de lingotes de oro. Después de descansar un día completo en la ciudad, estaba inquieto porque sabía que si la nota era cierta, a las 11:59 pm ya se había perdido un juego de oro. Al día siguiente, compró un camello y viajó al sitio en medio día. ¡La caja tenía otro juego de 24 lingotes de oro! Inmediatamente, estos fueron empacados en su bolso. Después de unas horas de descanso, volvió a despegar con su cansado camello. Como el camello no había descansado lo suficiente y se había llenado de agua, se derrumbó y murió a mitad de camino. Siguió caminando frenéticamente hacia la ciudad para volver a probar el oro. ¡Sí! ¡Son reales! Ahora, necesitaba dejarlos en algún lugar y volver por más. El hombre decidió comprar una gran granja semi abandonada para enterrar los lingotes de oro en un lugar aislado cerca del granero. Compró una caravana de camellos, víveres, jarras de agua, alimento seco y equipo de protección contra el intenso calor con el propósito de proteger a los camellos. Una vez que llegó a la zona desierta, acampó con la intención de quedarse un mes y recolectar la mayor cantidad de oro posible. Recogió un total de 720 lingotes de oro y estaba listo para regresar a la granja. Una vez en la granja, los enterró junto con los demás. Descansó un día e inmediatamente repitió el proceso. Compró camellos frescos y viajó a la zona desierta para recolectar más lingotes de oro. Pasó los últimos años de su vida repitiendo viajes, recolectando lingotes de oro, regresando a la granja, enterrándolos y regresando por más. A pesar de ser inmensamente rico, nunca compró nada más que suministros y camellos para los múltiples viajes. Nunca invirtió el oro, compró propiedades, donó a los necesitados o simplemente cambió parte de él en moneda para obtener un retorno de su inversión. Todo el oro simplemente fue enterrado bajo tierra, nada salió de él.*

Author: Roberto Swazo

*Cultural Hints*

In some cultures, the idea of individual goals is not quite accepted or embraced. Instead, there are collective goals that are sought after and reflect a sense of belonging to something bigger than oneself. Perhaps the challenge for the counselor is how to "promote" the idea of self-development as an independent unit with the intent of benefiting the group through personal investment. This could be translated into achieving the highest academic degree possible, applying for high paying jobs, competing in individual sports with the idea of earning Olympic medals, and similar individual objectives that can be achieved and converted into group achievements.

**Processing questions for the clients (Preguntas de proceso para los/as clientes)**

1.  What is your initial impression about this microfiction? What would you say about the main character? Explain. (*¿Cuál es tu impresión inicial sobre esta microficción? ¿Qué dirías del personaje principal? Explicar.*)
2.  Each one of the gold ingots out of the 24 that were given every day represent an hour of your life. After a day is over, the 24 hours of life given to you are lost and you are given another 24 hours again. The main character was given the chance to use each one of the gold ingots with a purpose. He decided not to invest in them as he did not have a goal in mind. Therefore, he used the remainder of his life to get more "free" gold ingots (equivalent to hours of life) to hide them. The main question is, what are you doing with each hour

of your life? How are you investing these hours given to you and what goal is directing these hours of activity provided to you? Be honest with yourself, and articulate a summary of your hours and which ones of these are guided by specific goals. (*Cada uno de los 24 lingotes de oro que se entregan todos los días representa una hora de tu vida. Después de que termina un día, las 24 horas de vida que se te otorgaron se pierden y se te otorgan otras 24 horas nuevamente. Al personaje principal se le dio la oportunidad de usar cada uno de los lingotes de oro con un propósito. Decidió no invertir en ellos porque no tenía un objetivo en mente. Por lo tanto, utilizó el resto de su vida para conseguir más lingotes de oro "gratis" (equivalentes a horas de vida) para esconderlos. La pregunta principal es, ¿qué estás haciendo con cada hora de tu vida? ¿Cómo estás invirtiendo estas horas que se te otorgan y qué objetivo dirige estas horas de actividad que se te brindan? Se honesto/a contigo mismo/a y articula un resumen de tus horas y cuál de ellas está guiada por objetivos específicos.*)

3.  Observe the picture that follows. Each step on the staircase represents an action guided by a short-term goal that is leading you to a long-term goal. You determine the long-term goal or what is generally making you move forward. Are you able to identify at least three or four long-term goals in your life? Can you label them on the picture as well as the short-term goals leading to it? Process and create a self-talk dialogue to ensure that these are rational and positive goals. (*Cada paso en la escalera representa una acción guiada por una meta a corto plazo que te lleva a una meta a largo plazo. Tú determinas la meta a largo plazo o lo que generalmente te hace avanzar. Observa la imagen de abajo. ¿Puedes identificar al menos de tres a cuatro metas a largo plazo en tu vida? ¿Puedes etiquetarlos*

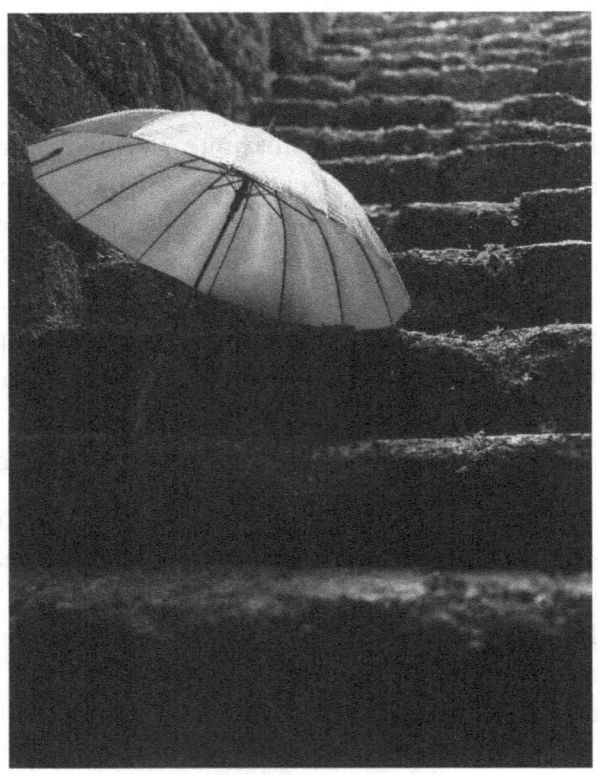

*Figure 16.1* Climbing Stairs

*en la imagen, así como los objetivos a corto plazo que los conducen? Procesa y crea un diálogo interno para asegurarse de que estos sean objetivos racionales y positivos.)*

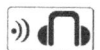 **Sayings (*dichos*)**

 *Saying #1*

"Animals wander around in circles in the wilderness looking for food and shelter. You got both, why are you still wandering in circles?"

*"Los animales deambulan en círculos por el desierto en busca de alimento y refugio. Tienes ambos, ¿por qué sigues dando vueltas en círculos?"*

Author: Mizrahi Hebrew saying (S. Mordechai, personal communication, July 7, 2021).

 **Processing questions for the clients (Preguntas de proceso para los/as clientes)**

1. There is a contextual message about wandering in the wilderness for food gathering and shelter. How would you interpret this? Explain. (*Hay un mensaje contextual sobre vagar por el desierto en busca de comida y refugio. ¿Cómo interpretarías esto? Explicar.*)

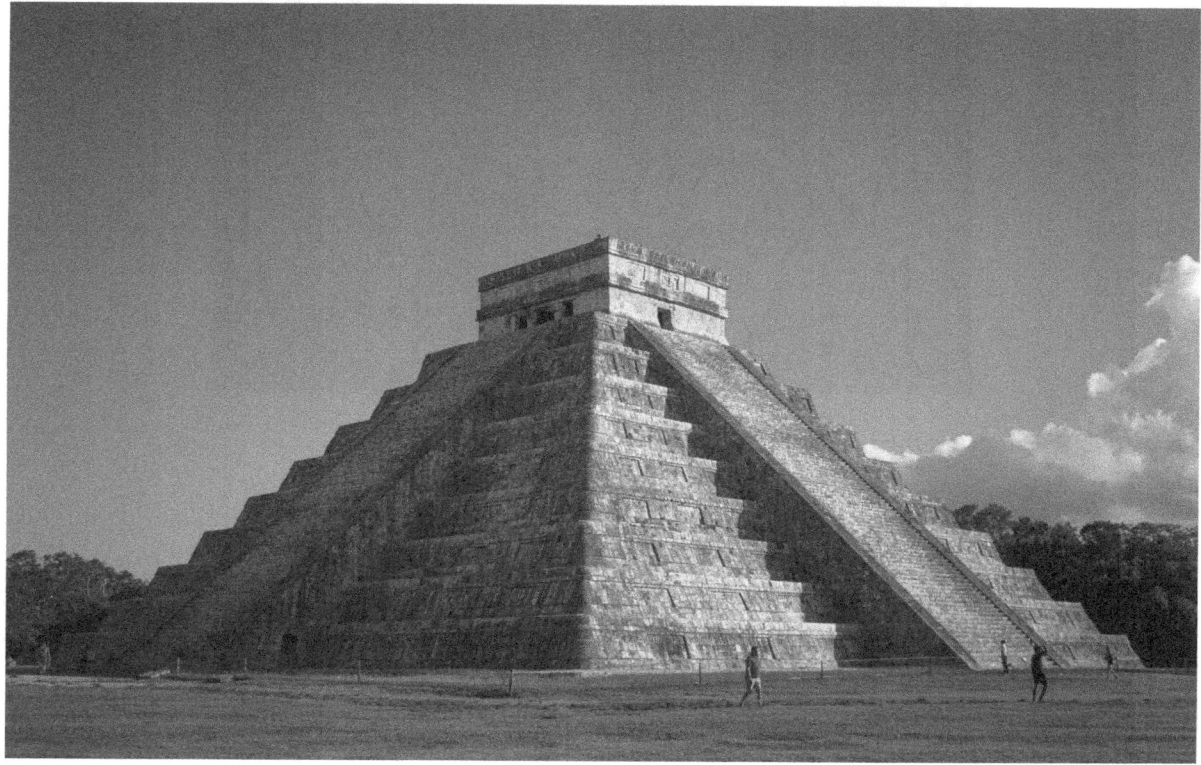

*Figure 16.2* Hierarchy of Needs

2. Analyze the pyramid that follows as described by Maslow. Where are you at this precise moment? What is lacking and why? What is currently impeding you to escalate to the next level/s? Describe. (*Analiza la pirámide a continuación como lo describe Maslow.*

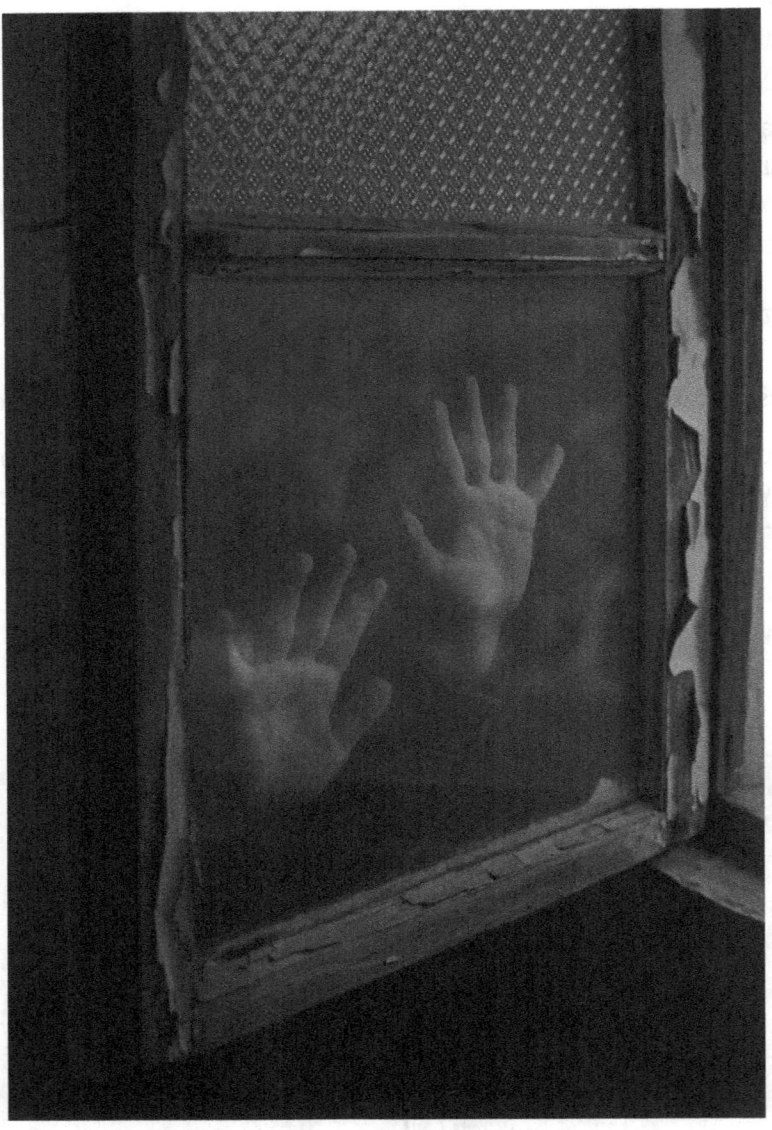

*Figure 16.3* Hands on the Inside of a Window

   *¿Dónde estás en este preciso momento? ¿Qué falta y por qué? ¿Qué te impide actualmente escalar al siguiente nivel? Describir.*)

3. Analyze the picture that follows and describe how it resembles you and at what specific points of your life. Elaborate. (*Analiza la imagen de abajo y describe en qué se parece a ti y en qué momentos específicos de tu vida. Elaborar.*)

*Saying #2*

"The goal is the beginning of today."
*"La meta es el principio de hoy."*

Author: Unknown (Goal Quotes, 2021).

 **Processing questions for the clients (Preguntas de proceso para los/as clientes)**

1. Interpret this quote based on TODAY. Is this day a result of a short-term, long-term, professional, personal, financial, business, or career goal? Is this day a result of a health/fitness or lifetime goal? Produce some specifics. (*Interpreta esta cita basada en HOY. ¿Es este día el resultado de un objetivo a corto, largo plazo, profesional o personal, financiero, empresarial o profesional? ¿Es este día el resultado de una meta de salud/forma física o de por vida? Produce detalles al respecto.*)

2. How do you feel at the end of a day, week, month, or year? What mechanisms are you using to evaluate growth and development? Elaborate. (*¿Cómo te sientes al final de un día, semana, mes o año? ¿Qué mecanismos estás utilizando para evaluar el crecimiento y el desarrollo? Elaborar.*)

3. ***Strength bombardment technique.*** Before the beginning of a week find the following: (***Técnica de bombardeo de fuerza.*** *Antes del comienzo de una semana, busque lo siguiente:*)

   a. A daily quote with a positive message related to goal achievement. (*Una cita diaria con un mensaje positivo relacionado con la consecución de objetivos.*)

   b. A spiritual message from any religious orientation that enhances your focus and drives you to be a better person. (*Un mensaje espiritual de cualquier orientación religiosa que mejora tu enfoque y te impulsa a ser una mejor persona.*)

   c. A piece of music that inspires you to move forward and accomplish your goals. (*Una pieza musical que te inspira a seguir adelante y lograr tus objetivos.*)

   d. A piece of art that inspires you and engages the non-cognitive part of you and nourishes the emotional intelligence toward goal completion. (*Una obra de arte que te inspira y compromete tu parte no cognitiva y nutre la inteligencia emocional hacia la consecución de la meta.*)

 **Quotes**

 *Quote #1*

"If you do what you have always done, you will achieve what you have always achieved."
*"Si haces lo que siempre has hecho, conseguirás lo que siempre has conseguido."*

Tony Robbins. He is an American motivational speaker and writer (2021).

**Processing questions for the clients (Preguntas de proceso para los/as clientes)**

1. Routine has its advantages if it is a productive and regenerative process. However, there are routines that lead to mediocrity, boredom, and stagnation. Complete the following table:

   (*La rutina tiene sus ventajas si se trata de un proceso productivo y regenerativo. Sin embargo, hay rutinas que conducen a la mediocridad, el aburrimiento y el estancamiento. Completa la siguiente tabla:*)

   *Table 16.1* Examining Routines to Explore Productivity

| Make a list of your daily routines. Include ALL of them, even the most mundane ones! (*Haz una lista de tus rutinas diarias. ¡Incluye TODAS, incluso las más mundanas!*) | How long have you been performing these routines? Try to be as specific as possible. (*¿Cuánto tiempo llevas realizando estas rutinas? Trata de ser lo más específico posible.*) | Did you come up with these routines or are these learned from someone else? (*¿Se te ocurrieron estas rutinas o las aprendiste de otra persona?*) | Rate each routine as productive, neutral, or counterproductive. How do you know that this self-rating process is accurate? (*Califica cada rutina como productiva, neutral y contraproducente. ¿Cómo sabes que este proceso de autoevaluación es preciso?*) | What can you do to readapt the neutral and counterproductive ones into productivity? (*¿Qué puedes hacer para readaptar los neutrales y contraproducentes a la productividad?*) |
|---|---|---|---|---|
| 1. | | | | |
| 2. | | | | |
| 3. | | | | |
| 4. | | | | |
| 5. | | | | |

2. *Self-talk technique*. Engage yourself in a constant self-analysis process for at least a week in order to find cognitive or thought processes that are sabotaging your personal growth and development. For instance, attempt to track your thought processes while performing monotonous tasks or things that you do routinely. As Tony Robbins says: "*If you do what you have always done, you will achieve what you have always achieved.*" Then, notice what irrational thoughts are being planted in your mind by yourself or others that are affecting your ability to execute your goals and daily activities leading to a different outcome. Write them on a piece of paper and don't let these escape your short-term memory. Find ways to dispute these irrational thoughts or messages and substitute them with positive and nourishing ones.

   (*Técnica de diálogo interno. Comprométete en un proceso de autoanálisis constante durante al menos una semana para encontrar procesos cognitivos o de pensamiento que están saboteando tu crecimiento y desarrollo personal. Por ejemplo, intenta rastrear tus procesos de pensamiento mientras realizas tareas monótonas o cosas que haces de forma rutinaria. Como dice el autor de la cita: "Si haces lo que siempre has hecho, lograrás lo que siempre has logrado". Entonces, ¿qué pensamientos irracionales están siendo plantados en tu mente por ti mismo o por otros que están afectando tu capacidad de ejecución? Tus objetivos y actividades diarias conducen a un resultado diferente. Escríbelos en una hoja de papel y no permitas que se escapen de tu memoria a corto plazo. Encuentra formas de disputar estos pensamientos o mensajes irracionales y sustitúyelos por otros positivos y enriquecedores.)*

3. ***Magic wand technique.*** If you could change one thing TODAY in order to prevent what you typically do and help you achieve what you really would like to do, what would it be and how does it look? What is preventing you from doing it? Is it out of reach or is it a matter of adjusting your lifestyle? Explain.

   (***Técnica de varita mágica.*** *¿Si pudieras cambiar una cosa HOY para evitar lo que normalmente haces y ayudarte a lograr lo que realmente te gustaría hacer? ¿Qué sería y cómo luce? ¿Qué te impide hacerlo? ¿Está fuera de tu alcance o se trata de ajustar tu estilo de vida? Explicar.)*

## Quote #2

"Successful and unsuccessful people don't vary much in their abilities. They vary in their desires to reach their potential."

   *"Las personas exitosas y no exitosas no varían mucho en sus habilidades. Varían en sus deseos para alcanzar su potencial."*

Author: John Maxwell. He is an American author, speaker, and pastor who has written several books, primarily focusing on leadership (2011).

## Processing questions for the clients (Preguntas de proceso para los/as clientes)

1. What is the meaning of this quote? Explain. (*¿Cuál es el significado de esta cita? Explicar.*)
2. What is the difference between a wish and a goal? Provide an example and elaborate. (*¿Cuál es la diferencia entre un deseo y una meta? Da un ejemplo y elabora.*)
3. Watch the following video about how to set goals and how to achieve them. Take notes and create a master plan that includes weekly, monthly, and yearly goals. This takes time and real dedication but it will dictate the degree of success that you will achieve. You must be specific and make sure that you rank these goals in the following categories: short-term, long-term, professional, personal, financial, business, career, health/fitness, and lifetime goals.

   www.youtube.com/watch?v=GOfl2sbgPhk

   (*Mira el siguiente video sobre cómo establecer metas y cómo lograrlas. Toma notas y crea un plan maestro que incluya metas semanales, mensuales y anuales. Esto requiere tiempo y dedicación real, pero determinará el grado de éxito que alcanzarás. Debes ser específico y asegurarte de clasificar estos objetivos en las siguientes categorías: a corto plazo, a largo plazo, objetivo profesional o personal, objetivo financiero, comercial o profesional, salud/estado físico y objetivos de por vida.) www.youtube.com/watch?v=GHI8eU10pKY*

### ·)) 🎧 Quote #3

"It doesn't matter where you come from. What matters is where you are going."
*"No importa de dónde vengas. Lo que importa es a dónde vas."*

Author: Brian Tracy. He is a Canadian-American motivational public speaker and self-development author (2021).

### ·)) 🎧 Processing questions for the clients (Preguntas de proceso para los/as clientes)

1. Attempt to provide a personal interpretation of this quote and contextualize it to your current situation. Explain. (*Intenta proporcionar una interpretación personal de esta cita y contextualizarla a tu situación actual. Explicar.*)
2. Take out a sheet of paper and draw five concentric circles to place the following within each one of them. For purposes of this exercise, the closer that you are to the inner circle or center, the more important these goals are to you: (*Dibuje cinco circulos concéntricos para colocar lo siguiente dentro de cada uno de ellos. Para los propósitos de este ejercicio, cuanto más cerca esté del círculo interno o del centro, más importantes serán estos objetivos para ti:*)

   - personal goals. (*metas personales.*)
   - health/fitness goals. (*metas de salud y aptitud física.*)
   - career/business goals. (*metas de carreras y negocios.*)
   - financial goals. (*metas financieras.*)
   - spiritual goals. (*metas espirituales.*)
   - personal relationships goals. (*metas de relaciones personales.*)
   - family oriented goals. (*metas orientadas a la familia.*)
   - leisure activities goals. (*metas de actividades de ocio.*)

Once you have completed the labeling of the concentric circles, answer the following questions: (*Una vez que hayas completado el etiquetado de los círculos concéntricos, responde a las siguientes preguntas:*)

- What motivates you to place one set of goals over another? (*¿Qué te motiva a colocar un conjunto de objetivos sobre otro?*)
- What are the implications of changing one set of goals over the other? (*¿Cuáles son las implicaciones de cambiar un conjunto de objetivos sobre el otro?*)
- If you were to compare ALL your life activities from last year, what does it say about the current ranking of these goals? (*Si tuvieras que comparar TODAS las actividades de tu vida del año pasado, ¿qué dice sobre la clasificación actual de estos objetivos?*)
- Elaborate on each one of them. (*Elabora en cada uno de estos.*)

3.  The great Spanish painter Salvador Dali said that "no masterpiece was created by a lazy artist." And, Stephen Covey, the American author of the *Seven Habits of Highly Effective People*, said that "everything that we do in life should start with the end in mind." What key principles can you extract from these two short quotes? Additionally, how much of your current way of achieving any type of personal, professional, spiritual, or health/fitness goal is based on a short spur of energy that fades away with time or in the absence of an immediate outcome? And, how can you create a more systematic strategy to overcome these obstacles?

    (*El gran pintor español Salvador Dalí dijo que "ninguna obra maestra fue creada por un artista perezoso". Y Stephen Covey, el autor estadounidense de Seven Habits of Highly Effective People dijo que "todo lo que hacemos en la vida debe comenzar con el final en mente". ¿Qué principios claves puedes extraer de estas dos breves citas? Además, ¿cuánto de tu forma actual de lograr cualquier tipo de objetivo personal, profesional, espiritual o de salud/condición física se basa en un breve impulso de energía que se desvanece con el tiempo o en ausencia de un resultado inmediato? Y, ¿cómo puedes crear una estrategia más sistemática para superar estos obstáculos?*)

## References

Goal Quotes. (2021, August 23). https://quotefancy.com/goal-quotes

Maxwell, J. C. (2011). *The Maxwell Daily Reader: 365 Days of insight to develop the leader within you and influence those around you.* Thomas Nelson.

Robbins, T. (2021, June 15). www.goodreads.com/quotes/36479-if-you-do-what-you-ve-always-done-you-ll-get-what

Tracy, B. (2021, May 13). www.goodreads.com/author/quotes/22033.Brian_Tracy

# 17 Future

According to the Merriam-Webster Dictionary (n.d.), future is defined as: (a) time that is to come, (b) what is going to happen, and (c) an expectation of advancement or progressive development. The concept of future is defined differently by many individuals and has somewhat of a subjective meaning or connotation. If one had to survey random individuals off the street about what the future is going to look like some will have answers such as: we will have space stations in different planets, moon bases, some sort of undersea cities, wealthy people will have personal submarines, maybe hover cars will be the norm, jetpacks will be used for traveling short distances, space travel will be as routine as taking an airplane, people will have video phones that will transmit smells and sensations, most middle class individuals will have humanoid robot servants, there will be cures for cancer and all kinds of other diseases and the world will be free of illnesses, poverty will be eradicated, there will be one controlling government, death will be conquered and immortality will be achieved, since there is one government all countries will cease to engage in wars, and happiness will be achieved. Of course, others would be more pessimistic and would see these with negative lenses and different twists.

What is fascinating about these types of questions is that most of the time we refuse to break down the concept of the future into manageable pieces that apply directly to our current lives. For instance, the future can be broken down into small intervals that would specifically apply to our mundane lifestyles. And of course, the future is as elusive as the present and the past, as all of these are constructs that are intertwined and at times difficult to measure. Therefore, the concept of time in counseling and psychotherapy is viewed as intervals of space that lead to actions between distinctive events. For example, "I will do x or y between breakfast and lunch or between lunch and dinner." Or, "I will devote my time to performing x or y tasks between the time that I start my stopwatch and the time that it stops with an alarm." Moreover, "I will stop performing a negative activity (i.e., smoking, drinking excessively, thinking negatively) from the beginning of the month and will evaluate my performance at the end of the month." The concept of time and more specifically the future within time is a critical construct that is used to set goals in anticipation of changes in behaviors, emotions, or thoughts as a result of the psychotherapeutic interventions. Hence, the construct of the future is of extreme importance because it shows progress, regression, or stagnation in our clients.

See also: goals, inspiration, motivation, identity, and liberation

DOI: 10.4324/9781003145943-21

## Cultural Hints

The concept of time is very fluid in many cultures and there is not necessarily a clear distinction between past, present, and future because there is a flow of life that is conceptualized cyclically. For instance, in most Native American cultures, events from hundreds of years ago are reported as if they occurred recently. Similarly, in Asian cultures, the presence of ancestors who died centuries ago is felt as a concurrent event as their memories are remembered almost daily by lighting candles and saying a prayer. Thus, there is a present communication with ancestors who passed away a long time ago but who have an inherent presence in today's activities.

## Microfiction

### I Can Hold the Future in My Hands

Since elementary school, life has been like a race for Liz. She had been working and studying non-stop since she could recall. She always knew exactly what she wanted to do with her life and how to get there. For instance, while she was in 5th grade, she started studying very hard to be in the best program upon advancing to middle school. She spent sleepless nights reading all kinds of books and completing various mathematics and sciences pamphlets. Certainly, she was accepted in the advanced courses in 6th grade and she already had her mind set on completing middle school with top honors in order to enter high school as a path to college. Liz always got inspired by successful women who were wealthy, intelligent, and highly educated. She was mesmerized by the lifestyle of the educated and wealthy and all the things that they could have in life. She knew that the only way that she could get there was by using her intellectual abilities in order to succeed in life. Then, she finished middle school and high school among the top 3 students in class. While she kept a full study load, she was able to hold a part-time job and save money for college. In essence, Liz could not enjoy the perks of high school life because she had no time for things that were not going to help her achieve her dreams for the future. She did not date anyone or have a romantic relationship. Her social life was practically nonexistent. Once she entered college, she had a part-time job at a business agency that helped her pay her bills and part of her college expenses and tuition. She was working and studying frantically while keeping her eyes on the ultimate goal of being a successful woman who at some point in the future was going to retire wealthy and comfortably. Once again, there was no time for a social life during college as she was focused on completing her degree. She used to say: "one day, once I finish college, I will get a great job, a spouse, and my own property." Finally, she finished her bachelor's degree! She thought that this was going to bring some inner peace and a sense of achievement, but it did not. Also, she did not have time to celebrate this achievement, as she needed to apply for jobs! After multiple interviews, she was selected for a top position. Immediately, she started working extra hours in order to pay off her college tuition debt. Right after this, she purchased a small apartment and her first new car. After a couple of years of intense work, she met Carl. They married and bought a house. Now she had to work harder to pay off the mortgage and other debts. She still had her eyes on the final goal, retiring wealthy and comfortable. After a couple of years, they had their first child, then, they bought a bigger house and a van, and started a college fund for the kid. Long hours of work and barely time for her family was her lifestyle; however, she had her eyes on the ultimate goal! She decided to complete an MBA in order to get a promotion in the agency. After many sleepless nights, exams, and challenges, Liz completed the degree and was rapidly promoted to a CEO position. Now, she had more responsibilities, less family time, and less of a social life. However, her eyes were on the final goal! She and Carl had another child, more responsibilities, and no family life. Liz was determined to save, invest, and retire early. Long story short, after working, working, and working like a farm animal without any respite, Liz and Carl achieved their financial goal. She could retire at 62 and spend the rest of her days playing golf in the sunny coast of Florida. Liz and Carl sold their properties and purchased an apartment close to the golf course. She said, finally I can reap the rewards of my work and efforts, finally! Two months later after moving to Florida, and not having even one weekend off since high school, Liz had a massive heart attack that killed her instantly.

(Español)

 ## Microficción

### *Puedo Tener el Futuro en mis Manos*

*Desde la escuela primaria, la vida ha sido como un auto de carreras para Liz. Había estado trabajando y estudiando sin parar desde que tenía memoria. Siempre supo exactamente lo que quería hacer con su vida y cómo llegar allí. Por ejemplo, mientras estaba en quinto grado, comenzó a estudiar muy duro para estar en el mejor programa al avanzar a la escuela secundaria. Pasó noches sin dormir leyendo todo tipo de libros y completando varios folletos de matemáticas y ciencias. Ciertamente, fue aceptada en los cursos avanzados en sexto grado y ya tenía la mente puesta en completar la escuela secundaria con los máximos honores para poder ingresar a la escuela secundaria como un camino a la universidad. Liz siempre se inspiró en mujeres exitosas que eran ricas, inteligentes y con un alto nivel de educación. Estaba hipnotizada por el estilo de vida de los ricos y educados y todas las cosas que podrían tener en la vida. Sabía que la única forma de llegar allí era utilizando sus habilidades intelectuales para tener éxito en la vida. Luego, terminó la escuela media y secundaria entre los 3 mejores estudiantes de la clase. Si bien mantuvo una carga completa de estudios, pudo tener un trabajo de medio tiempo y ahorrar dinero para la universidad. En esencia, Liz no podía disfrutar de las ventajas de la vida en la escuela secundaria porque no tenía tiempo para cosas que no la ayudarían a lograr sus sueños para el futuro. Ella no salía con nadie ni tuvo una relación romántica. Su vida social era prácticamente inexistente. Una vez que ingresó a la universidad, tuvo un trabajo de medio tiempo en una agencia de negocios que la ayudó a pagar sus facturas y parte de sus gastos universitarios y de matrícula. Trabajaba y estudiaba frenéticamente mientras mantenía sus ojos en el objetivo final de ser una mujer exitosa que en algún momento en el futuro se jubilaría rica y cómodamente. Una vez más, no hubo tiempo para una vida social durante la universidad, ya que estaba concentrada en completar su título. Ella solía decir: "un día, una vez que termine la universidad, obtendré un gran trabajo, un cónyuge y mi propia propiedad". ¡Finalmente, terminó su licenciatura! Ella pensó que esto iba a traer algo de paz interior y una sensación de logro, pero no fue así. Sin embargo, no tuvo tiempo para celebrar este logro, ¡necesitaba postularse para trabajos!*

*Después de múltiples entrevistas, fue seleccionada para un puesto superior. Inmediatamente, comenzó a trabajar horas extra para pagar su deuda de matrícula universitaria. Inmediatamente después de esto, compró un pequeño departamento y su primer auto nuevo. Después de un par de años de intenso trabajo, conoció a Carl.*

*Se casaron y compraron una casa. Ahora tenía que trabajar más duro para pagar la hipoteca y otras deudas. Todavía tenía los ojos puestos en el objetivo final, jubilarse rica y cómoda. Después de un par de años, tuvieron su primer hijo, luego compraron una casa más grande, una camioneta y comenzaron un fondo universitario para el niño. Largas horas de trabajo y apenas tiempo para su familia era su estilo de vida, sin embargo, ¡tenía los ojos puestos en el objetivo final!*

*Ella y Carl tuvieron otro hijo, más responsabilidades y ninguna vida familiar. Liz estaba decidida a ahorrar, invertir y jubilarse antes de tiempo. En pocas palabras, después de trabajar, trabajar y trabajar como un animal de granja sin ningún respiro, Liz y Carl lograron su objetivo financiero. Podría retirarse a los 62 años y pasar el resto de sus días jugando al golf en la soleada costa de Florida. Liz y Carl vendieron sus propiedades y compraron un apartamento cerca del campo de golf. Ella dijo, ¡finalmente puedo cosechar las recompensas de mi trabajo y esfuerzos, finalmente! Dos meses más tarde, después de mudarse a Florida, y sin tener ni un fin de semana libre desde la escuela secundaria, Liz tuvo un ataque cardíaco masivo que la mató instantáneamente.*

Author: Roberto Swazo.

## Processing questions for the clients (Preguntas de proceso para los/as clientes)

1. What is your visceral reaction after reading this microfiction? What kind of emotions does this story evoke in you? Elaborate. (*¿Cuál es tu reacción visceral después de leer esta microficción? ¿Qué tipo de emociones te evoca esta historia? Elaborar.*)

2. Can you explain what happened to Liz's life and what was the critical issue that she faced? What do you think was her internal struggle about? Discuss. (*¿Puedes explicar qué pasó con la vida de Liz y cuál fue el problema crítico que enfrentó? ¿De qué crees que fue su lucha interna? Discutir.*)

3. Can you relate to her character? If not, have you ever seen anyone close to you who resembles Liz's story? What can you learn from this person? Explain. (*¿Puedes identificarte con su personaje? Si no es así, ¿alguna vez has visto a alguien cercano a ti que se parezca a la historia de Liz? ¿Qué puedes aprender de esta persona? Explicar.*)

## Sayings (*dichos*)

### *Saying #1*

"Fools speak of the past, wise men of the present, and madmen of the future."
*"Los tontos hablan del pasado, los sabios del presente y los locos del futuro."*

Author: Napoleon Bonaparte was a French military and political leader who rose to prominence during the French Revolution and led several successful campaigns during the Revolutionary Wars (*Aphorisms and Thoughts*, 2018).

**Processing questions for the clients (Preguntas de proceso para los/as clientes)**

1.  In a nutshell, how do you break down this quote? And, can you provide an illustration related to your own life? Discuss.

    (*En pocas palabras, ¿cómo se desglosa esta cita? Y, ¿puedes proporcionar una ilustración relacionada con tu propia vida? Discutir.*)

2.  There is obviously an intersection between some of the subconstructs of time (i.e., past, present, future), and we choose to embrace some of these more than others. What factor does the future play in your life and how does it look? Also, is your future shaping your current behaviors and emotions? In what way? Elaborate.

    (*Obviamente, existe una intersección entre algunos de los subconstructos del tiempo (es decir, pasado, presente, futuro), y elegimos abrazar algunos de estos más que otros. ¿Qué factor juega el futuro en tu vida y cómo se ve el mismo? Además, ¿tu futuro está dando forma a tus comportamientos y emociones actuales? ¿De qué manera? Elaborar.*)

3.  ***Empty chair technique (Gestalt theory).*** Place an empty chair in front of you. Then, decide which of the two subconstructs of time (i.e., past or present) you are representing while sitting in front of the empty chair. Then, the empty chair represents either the past or the present. What questions would you ask to yourself as you are looking at the past image of yourself? Interview yourself about what made you (in the past) make a series of decisions that you are paying the consequences for in the present and how these will affect the future? Finally, what does yourself in the future say about these dynamics and what can be changed now to alter the future? Provide details.

    [***Técnica de la silla vacía (teoría de la Gestalt).*** *Coloca una silla vacía frente a ti. Luego, decide cuál de las dos subconstructos del tiempo (es decir, pasado o presente) estás representando mientras estás sentado frente a la silla vacía. Entonces, la silla vacía representa el pasado o el presente. ¿Qué preguntas te harías a ti mismo mientras miras la imagen pasada de ti mismo? Entrevistarte sobre lo que le hiciste (en el pasado) y tomar una serie de decisiones por las que estás pagando las consecuencias en el presente y cómo éstas afectarán el futuro. Finalmente, ¿qué dices tú mismo/a en el futuro sobre estas dinámicas y qué se puede cambiar ahora para alterar el futuro? Proporcionar detalles.*]

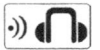 *Saying #2*

"It is better to have one bird in the hand rather than one hundred flying."
"*Más vale pájaro en mano que ciento volando.*"

Author: Unknown. Popular Latin American saying (*A Dictionary of Mexican American Proverbs*, 1987).

 **Processing questions for the clients (Preguntas de proceso para los/as clientes)**

1.  Put this quote in context and try to explain it based on your own experience or somebody else's experience. Explain.

    (*Pon esta cita en contexto e intenta explicarla según tu propia experiencia o la experiencia de otra persona. Explicar.*)

2. Take a look at the tree in the following photo. As you can see, it has bare branches. There are no leaves or fruits. Make small notes with dates (years) by each of the branches representing the things that you have aspired for in the future but have not materialized. It is probable that you have been thinking about all the permutations, angles, and complications of each one of these things that you have wanted in the future. It is most likely that a large number of them did not come to fruition. Sometimes trees are stripped from fresh branches, leaves, or fruits due to many factors such as droughts, insects, plagues, torrential rains, or animals that ate their leaves and some of the branches.

Can you determine which factors in your life affected the materialization of your future endeavors? Discuss.

(*Echa un vistazo al árbol de abajo. Como puedes ver, tiene ramas desnudas. No hay hojas ni frutos. Toma pequeñas notas con fechas (años) por cada una de las ramas que representan las cosas a las que has aspirado en el futuro pero no se han materializado. Es probable que hayas estado pensando en todas las permutaciones, ángulos y complicaciones de cada una de estas cosas que has querido en el futuro. Lo más probable es que una gran cantidad de ellas no se hayan materializado. A veces, los árboles son despojados de ramas, hojas o frutos frescos debido a muchos factores como sequías, insectos o plagas, lluvias torrenciales o animales que se comieron sus hojas y algunas de las ramas.*

*¿Puedes determinar qué factores de tu vida afectaron la materialización de tus futuros emprendimientos? Discutir.*)

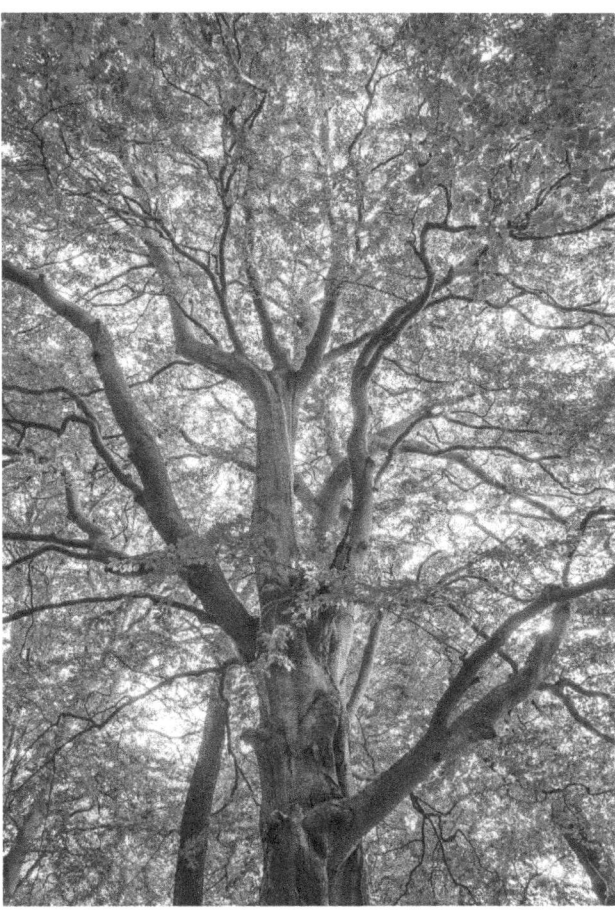

*Figure 17.1* Large Tree With Mostly Bare Branches

3. Lexy has remained unemployed for a long period of time because she has not found the ideal job that she wanted after completing her college education. She says that she is not going to "degrade herself by working on entry level jobs knowing that she has more potential than that." As a result, she is still living with her parents, disgruntled, and hoping to land the perfect job at some point. If you could talk to Lexy, what would you say to her? Now, how many times have you been on paralysis mode by waiting for the perfect conditions in order to act? Especially when you know that there are many opportunities "out there," however, none have materialized so far. Discuss.

*(Lexy ha permanecido desempleada durante un largo período de tiempo porque no ha encontrado el trabajo ideal que quería después de completar su educación universitaria. Ella dice que no se va a "degradar a sí misma trabajando en trabajos de nivel de entrada sabiendo que tiene más potencial que eso". Como resultado, todavía está con sus padres, disgustada y con la esperanza de conseguir el trabajo perfecto en algún momento. Si pudieras hablar con Lexy, ¿qué le dirías? Ahora bien, ¿cuántas veces has estado en modo de parálisis esperando las condiciones perfectas para actuar? Especialmente cuando sabes que hay muchas oportunidades "ahí fuera", sin embargo, ninguna se ha materializado hasta ahora. Discutir.)*

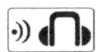 **Quotes**

 *Quote #1*

"The future belongs to those who believe in the beauty of their dreams."
*"El futuro pertenece a quienes creen en la belleza de sus sueños."*

Author: Eleanor Roosevelt (2017). She was an American political figure who served as a diplomat and activist. She served as the First Lady of the United States from March 4, 1933, to April 12, 1945, during her husband President Franklin D. Roosevelt's four terms in office, making her the longest-serving First Lady of the United States. In addition to being the First Lady, Eleanor Roosevelt served as United States Delegate to the United Nations General Assembly from 1945 to 1952.

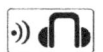 **Processing questions for the clients (Preguntas de proceso para los/as clientes)**

1. Do a quick search of Eleanor Roosevelt, explore her biography, and then attempt to explain the meaning of this quote based on her contextual reality and her contributions to the political and social landscapes of the US.

   *(Haz una búsqueda rápida de Eleanor Roosevelt, explora su biografía y luego intenta explicar el significado de esta cita en función de su realidad contextual y sus contribuciones a los paisajes políticos y sociales de los EE. UU.)*

2. ***Visual/guided imagery (mindfulness) technique.*** Close your eyes. Breathe in and breathe out. As you breathe, let the muscles in your neck and shoulders relax. Feel the tension going away and the heaviness of stress disappearing from your life. Forget about all the pressures of life, responsibilities, financial issues, and stressors of business or work. As

you do this, imagine a place that you have always loved to visit, be it a location, country, or a specific/special place. Or perhaps, imagine something that you have always wanted to have or a person that you would like to have a relationship with. Whatever it is, picture it mentally and do not let any thought disturb this image. Embrace it, feel it, touch it, and own it mentally. It is yours, it will happen, there is a mental certainty that this is a fact in your unique mental universe. After embracing it, slowly open your eyes, and describe the feelings of owning this image and how you can convert it into a reality.

(***Técnica de imágenes visuales/guiadas (Mindfulness).*** *Cierra tus ojos. Inhala y exhala. Mientras respiras, deja que los músculos del cuello y los hombros se relajen. Siente cómo la tensión desaparece y la pesadez del estrés desaparece de tu vida. Olvídate de todas las presiones de la vida, las responsabilidades, los problemas financieros y los factores estresantes de los negocios o el trabajo. Al hacer esto, imagina un lugar que siempre te ha gustado visitar, ya sea un lugar, un país o un lugar específico/especial. O quizás, imagina algo que siempre has querido tener o una persona con la que te gustaría tener una relación. Sea lo que sea, imagínala mentalmente y no permitas que ningún pensamiento perturbe esta imagen. Abrázalo, siéntelo, tócalo y sé dueño de él mentalmente. Es tuyo, sucederá, hay una certeza mental de que esto es un hecho en tu universo mental único. Después de abrazarla, abre lentamente los ojos y describe los sentimientos de poseer esta imagen y cómo puedes convertirla en realidad.*)

3. Looking forward to something good and positive in life can be a tremendous motivation to deal with the harsh reality of the present and the obstacles that we face. What is it that you are looking forward to in the future? What keeps you motivated and always looking to the light at the end of the tunnel? Explain.

(*Esperar algo bueno y positivo en la vida puede ser una tremenda motivación para lidiar con la dura realidad del presente y los obstáculos que enfrentamos. ¿Qué es lo que esperas en el futuro? ¿Qué te mantiene motivado y siempre mirando hacia la luz al final del túnel? Explicar.*)

 ## Quote #2

"Education is our passport to the future, for tomorrow belongs to the people who prepare for it today."

"*La educación es nuestro pasaporte hacia el futuro, porque el mañana pertenece a las personas que se preparan hoy.*"

Author: Malcolm X was an African American Muslim minister and human rights activist who was a popular figure during the civil rights movement (1964). He was a vocal spokesman for the Nation of Islam during the Civil Rights movement.

 **Processing questions for the clients (Preguntas de proceso para los/as clientes)**

1. What is the meaning of education according to this quote and how is the construct of the future intimately related to it? Explain.

*(¿Cuál es el significado de educación según esta cita y cómo se relaciona íntimamente con ella el constructo del futuro? Explicar.)*

2. There are various types of education. For instance, there is formal education involving the traditional route of K-12 and postsecondary education. Also, there is continuing education in which one takes additional courses in order to maintain a level of competence in a field. Additionally, there is the autodidactic education in which the individual acquires knowledge via the extraction of information from several resources in order to learn a craft or a vocation. Finally, there is the concept of education pertaining to learning for the pleasure of learning. All of them are closely related to the future. Are you able to place yourself within any of these types of education and how they have or could play a critical role in your future? Elaborate.

*(Hay varios tipos de educación. Por ejemplo, existe la educación formal que involucra la ruta tradicional de K-12 y educación postsecundaria. Además, hay educación continua en la que se toman cursos adicionales para mantener un nivel de competencia en un campo. Adicionalmente, está la educación autodidacta en la que el individuo adquiere conocimientos a través de la extracción de información de varios recursos para aprender un oficio o una vocación. Finalmente, está el concepto de educación que se refiere al aprendizaje por el placer de aprender. Todos ellos están estrechamente relacionados con el futuro. ¿Eres capaz de ubicarte en alguno de estos tipos de educación y cómo estos han tenido o podrían jugar un papel crítico en tu futuro? Elaborar.)*

3. **Deep breathing and meditation technique.** Close your eyes, relax your body, and start taking deep breaths in order to refocus your mind and your internal vision. Picture some type of goal that you have been trying to achieve for a long time. As you see this mental goal, break down mentally the educational steps needed to achieve it. Sustain some deep breathing patterns and maintain your mind free of any obstacles that could interfere with the crystallization of this goal. Maintain this process for no less than 20 minutes. Set a stopwatch in order to ensure that you have dedicated time to this exercise. Do not write down anything. For the next few days, repeat the process again. After a week, and after mastering the mental crystallization of this future goal that involves knowledge and education, take a piece of paper and write down the steps to achieve it. Now that it is on paper, you can read it and modify it. Do not act on it. For the next few days, engage in the deep breathing meditation process and read it again after completing each one of them. Now that this has been firmly established in your mind it is time to start operationalizing this future goal into manageable bits within the present. Attach timelines to each one of these manageable bits of present actions. Evaluate your actions on a weekly basis and later every month.

*(**Técnica de respiración profunda y meditación.** Cierra los ojos, relaja el cuerpo y comienza a respirar profundamente para enfocar tu mente y tu visión interna. Imagínate algún tipo de objetivo que has estado tratando de lograr durante mucho*

*tiempo. Al ver este objetivo mental, analiza mentalmente los pasos educativos necesarios para lograrlo. Mantén algunos patrones de respiración profunda y mantén tu mente libre de cualquier obstáculo que pueda interferir con la cristalización de este objetivo. Mantén este proceso durante no menos de 20 minutos. Configura un cronómetro para asegurarte de que has dedicado tiempo a este ejercicio. No escribas nada. Durante los próximos días, repite el proceso nuevamente. Pasada una semana, y después de dominar la cristalización mental de esta meta futura que involucra conocimiento y educación, toma un papel y escribe los pasos para lograrlo. Ahora que está en papel, puedes leerlo y modificarlo. No intentes hacerlo. Durante los próximos días, participa en el proceso de meditación de respiración profunda y léelo de nuevo después de completar cada uno de ellos. Ahora que esto se ha establecido firmemente en tu mente, es hora de comenzar a hacer operativa esta meta futura en partes manejables dentro del presente. Adjunta líneas de tiempo a cada una de estas partes manejables de acciones presentes. Evalúa tus acciones semanalmente y más tarde cada mes.)*

 ### Quote #3

3a. "You spend your whole life stuck in the labyrinth, thinking about how you'll escape one day, and how awesome it will be, and imagining that future keeps you going, but you never do it. You just use the future to escape the present."

3a. *"Pasas toda tu vida atrapado en el laberinto, pensando en cómo escaparás algún día y en lo maravilloso que será, e imaginando que el futuro te mantiene en marcha, pero nunca lo haces. Solo usa el futuro para escapar del presente."*

Author: John M. Green (2008). He is an American author and YouTube content creator. He won the 2006 Printz Award for his debut novel, *Looking for Alaska*, and his fourth solo novel, *The Fault in Our Stars*, debuted at number one on The New York Times Best Seller list in January 2012.

3b. "Why didn't I learn to treat everything like it was the last time? My greatest regret was how much I believed in the future."

3b. *"¿Por qué no aprendí a tratar todo como si fuera la última vez? Lo que más lamento es lo mucho que creía en el futuro."*

Author: Jonathan Safran Foer (2005). He is an American writer and novelist.

### Processing questions for the clients (Preguntas de proceso para los/as clientes)

1. See the picture of a labyrinth that follows. Describe it. What has been the labyrinth in your life? Provide specific details.

   (*Ve la imagen de un laberinto a continuación. Descríbelo. ¿Cuál ha sido el laberinto de tu vida? Proporciona detalles específicos.*)

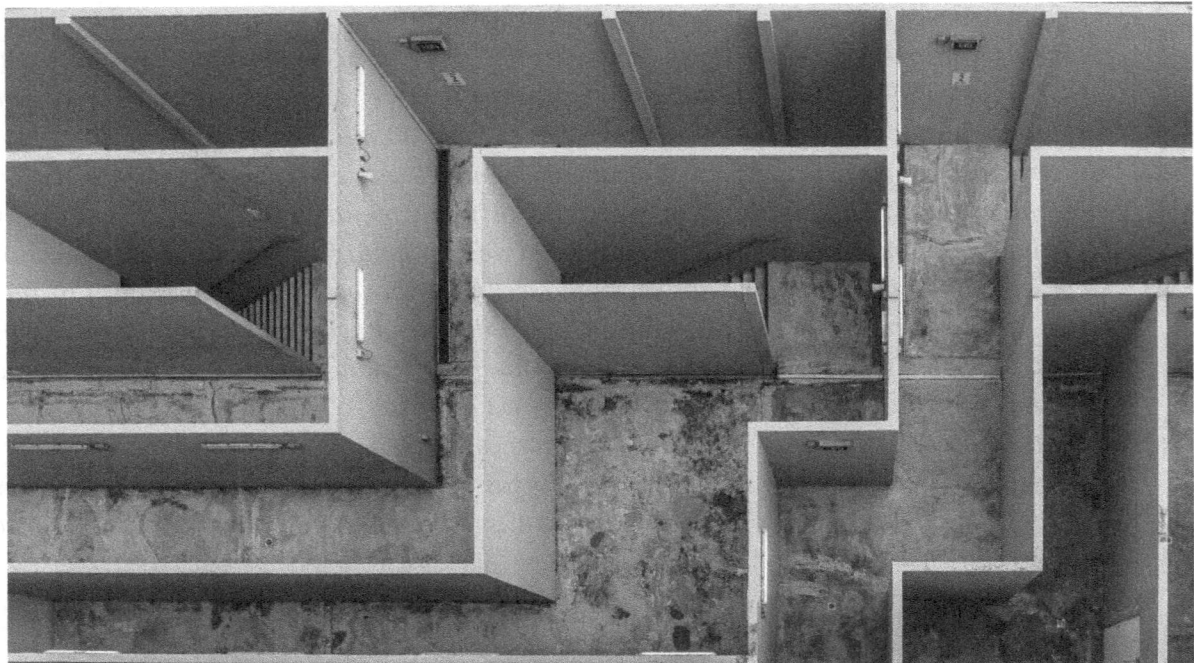

*Figure 17.2* Labyrinth

2. Take a big empty canvas and place it either on the floor or attach it to a wall. Use hand painting to represent what the future looks like to you. Even if you don't know how to draw or paint, the combination of colors or the amorphous shapes with intense or serene combinations will show what the future looks like to you. Do not feel constrained by any artistic limitation and simply let yourself express it all!

    (*Toma un lienzo grande y vacío y colócalo en el piso o colócalo en una pared. Usa pintura a mano para representar cómo se ve el futuro para ti. Aunque no sepas dibujar o pintar, la combinación de colores o las formas amorfas con combinaciones intensas o serenas te mostrarán cómo te depara el futuro. ¡No te sientas limitado por ninguna limitación artística y simplemente déjate expresar todo!*)

3. ***Reflective self-disclosure exercise.*** Look at the picture that follows. What does it say about the idea of reaching out for the stars while trying to keep the balance on a ladder? Stand in front of a mirror that allows you to see your face completely. Close your eyes and think about the stars that you are trying to reach and have "evaded you." Open your eyes, look deeply into your own eyes. And say this out loud: "Am I being honest with myself? Am I avoiding the present and not enjoying it while keeping the expectations that there is something better for me in the future in spite of the fact that I have never ever reached it?" Evaluate yourself, reflect, repeat, and reevaluate your ideas about the future and current activities. (***Ejercicio reflexivo de autorrevelación.*** *Mira la foto de abajo. ¿Qué dice sobre la idea de alcanzar la(s) estrella(s) mientras tratas de mantener el equilibrio en una escalera? Ponte de pie en frente a un espejo que te permita ver tu rostro por completo. Cierra los ojos y piensa en las estrellas que estás tratando de alcanzar y que te han "evadido". Abre*

*los ojos, mira profundamente en tus propios ojos. Y dilo en voz alta: "¿Estoy siendo honesto conmigo mismo? ¿Estoy evitando el presente y no disfrutándolo manteniendo las expectativas de que hay algo mejor para mí en el futuro a pesar de que nunca lo he alcanzado?" Evalúate, reflexiona, repite y reevalúa tus ideas sobre las actividades futuras y actuales.)*

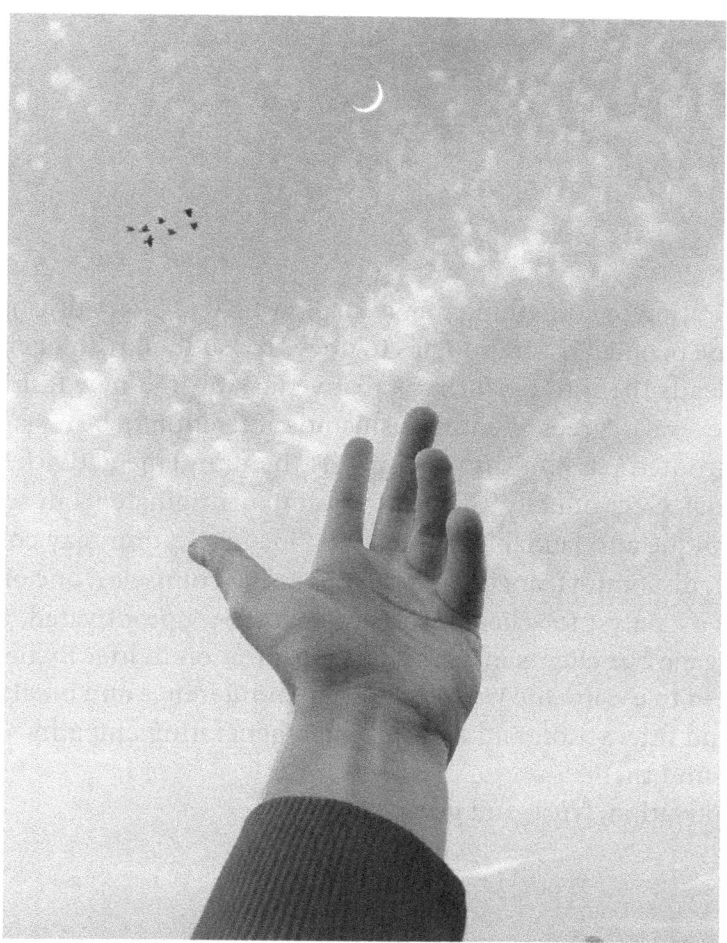

*Figure 17.3* Person's Hand Reaching for the Moon

## References

*Aphorisms and thoughts.* (2018). Alma Books.

*A dictionary of Mexican American proverbs.* (1987). Greenwood Press.

Foer, J. S. (2005). *Extremely loud and incredibly close.* Houghton Mifflin.

Green, J. (2008). *Looking for Alaska.* Penguin Young Readers Group.

Merriam-Webster. (n.d.). Future. In *Merriam-webster.com dictionary.* Retrieved June 18, 2021, from www.merriam-webster.com/dictionary/future

Roosevelt, E. (2017). My day July 4th, 1957. *The Eleanor Roosevelt papers digital edition.* https://www2.gwu.edu/~erpapers/myday/displaydoc.cfm?_y=1957&_f=md003845

X, M. (1964). *Malcolm's X speech at the foundation rally of the organization of Afro-American unity.* www.blackpast.org/african-american-history/speeches-african-american-history/1964-malcolm-x-s-speech-founding-rally-organization-afro-american-unity/

# 18 Inspiration

The concept of inspiration or something that is inspirational can vary drastically, according to each person. To some people, inspiration has to do with a sudden rush of energy, be it mental or emotional, that leads them to perform a creative task or in a new fashion. Inspiration is typically linked to several degrees of enthusiasm and motivation to be engaged to take action. It might be a deep-rooted passion that transcends the mundane activities and propels one forward toward a goal. Occasionally, the inspiration may originate from seeing others doing something that is unique and laudable. Sometimes this inspiration may come out of feelings of compassion, pain, discomfort, anger, or happiness. As a counselor, one of the greatest challenges is to serve as a catalyst for clients who are apathetic, unmotivated, unconcerned, and indifferent. Why engage our clients in a search for inspiration in life? By helping them in this search, we allow them to escape the walls of internal indifference and break into the reality of social connection and interaction and a by-product, generating empathy and care for themselves and those around them.

See also: hope, motivation, trust, and goals

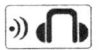 **Microfiction**

### Under the Blankets

On most winter days in St. Petersburg, Russia, it was cold and gray. People were out and about conducting their daily activities. Fleeting looks, no eye contact, quick steps, just trying to buy what is needed for the day and going straight to the train station. Although fairly successful, I do not have a fire in me for anything in life. Sure, family, work, blah, blah. However, nothing drives me. I guess that I am just normally bored with life. For no special reason, I started to pay attention to the people around me. All of them were seemingly able-bodied and capable of achieving what they wanted. However, after taking the train all of my life and walking freely through the streets of the center, I noticed a couple of older and disabled people sitting in a corner covered by layers of dirty blankets with an old dog by their side serving as companionship and a natural heater. Like a strong magnet, I felt compelled to reach out to them and connect. "Excuse me gentlemen, I know that it is cold and you must be hungry as well. I do not want to offend you and dehumanize you but can I make you an offer?" Puzzled by the attention that was given to them, they hesitated but silently agreed. "I will give you some rubles and also, I will purchase

DOI: 10.4324/9781003145943-22

a hot meal for you if you are so kind as to answer some questions that I have for you, alright? Again, I am not bribing you or taking advantage of you, I mean it." With tired eyes full of pain and dignity that had abandoned them years ago, they agreed. "Where are you from, why are you on the streets asking for money, and what did you do in the past?" I timidly asked. Lifting the end of the blankets one said: "Young man, my brother and I lost our legs years ago in the Chechen war fighting for mother Russia. The government sends us a small check large enough to pay for our food but not for a roof over our heads. We were proud soldiers, people would admire us when we were young and strong. Now, we are social leftovers. People despise us as a repugnant nuisance. We have to hide from the police as they do not want us begging on the streets. We drag ourselves like snakes because we cannot walk like you. These are our possessions, blankets, cardboards, what we are wearing, and our beloved dog Vladi." He stopped them from talking and had an urge to cry; a strange feeling of grief overcame him. Immediately, he gave them all the cash he had in his wallet at the moment and ran to the closest restaurant and brought two warm meals. From that day on he brought a different friend or family member and made them listen to their story. Like an electric shock, an idea struck him. A foundation for homeless veterans!! A few years later, he secured funding for homeless shelters with showers and food, city ordinances for sidewalk ramps, reusable wheelchairs, and warming centers for the homeless in the winter. "Life will never be the same for these human beings on the streets and for me!!"

(*Español*)

 **Microficción**

### *Bajo las Cobijas*

*Como la mayoría de los días de invierno en San Petersburgo, Rusia, hacía frío y gris. La gente estaba fuera y realizando sus actividades diarias. Miradas fugaces, sin contacto visual, pasos rápidos, solo tratando de comprar lo que se necesita para el día e ir directamente a la estación de tren. Aunque bastante exitoso, no tengo un fuego en mí por nada en la vida. Seguro, familia, trabajo, bla, bla. Sin embargo, nada me impulsa. Supongo que normalmente estoy aburrido de la vida. Sin ninguna razón especial, comencé a prestar atención a las personas que me rodeaban. Todos ellos estaban capacitados y eran capaces de conseguir lo que querían. Sin embargo, después de tomar el tren toda mi vida y caminar libremente por las calles del centro, noté a una pareja de personas frágiles y discapacitadas sentadas en un rincón cubiertas por capas de mantas sucias con un perro viejo a su lado sirviendo de compañía y un calentador natural. Como un imán fuerte, me sentí obligado a acercarme a ellos y conectarme. "Disculpe caballero, sé que hace frío y usted debe tener hambre también. No quiero ofenderte y deshumanizarte pero ¿puedo hacerte una oferta? Desconcertados por la atención que se les prestó, dudaron pero aceptaron en silencio. "Te daré algunos escombros y también, te compraré una comida caliente si eres tan amable de responder algunas preguntas que tengo para ti, ¿de acuerdo? Una vez más, no te estoy sobornando ni aprovechándome de ti, lo digo en serio". Con los ojos cansados llenos de dolor y dignidad que los había abandonado años atrás, estuvieron de acuerdo. "¿De dónde eres, por qué andas en la calle pidiendo dinero y qué solías hacer en el pasado?", Le pregunté tímidamente. Levantando el extremo de las mantas, uno dijo: "joven, mi hermano y yo perdimos las piernas hace años en la guerra de Chechenia luchando por la madre Rusia. El gobierno nos envía un pequeño cheque lo suficientemente grande para pagar nuestra comida, pero no para un techo sobre nuestras cabezas. Éramos soldados orgullosos, la gente nos admiraba cuando éramos jóvenes y fuertes. Ahora, somos sobras sociales. La gente nos desprecia como una molestia repugnante. Tenemos que escondernos de la policía porque no quieren que mendiguemos en las calles. Nos arrastramos como serpientes porque no podemos caminar como tú. Estas son nuestras posesiones, mantas, cartones, lo que llevamos puesto y nuestro querido perro Vladi". Les impidió hablar y sintió ganas de llorar; un extraño sentimiento de dolor se apoderó de él. Inmediatamente, les dio todo el dinero que tenía en su billetera en ese momento y corrió al restaurante más cercano y trajo dos comidas calientes. A partir de ese día trajo a un amigo o familiar diferente y les hizo escuchar su historia. Como una descarga eléctrica, se le ocurrió una idea. ¡Una fundación para veteranos sin hogar! Unos años más tarde, obtuvo fondos para refugios para personas sin hogar con duchas y comida, ordenanzas de la ciudad para rampas en las aceras, sillas de ruedas reutilizables y centros de calentamiento para personas sin hogar en el invierno. "¡La vida nunca será la misma para estos seres humanos en las calles y para mí!"*

Author: Roberto Swazo.

 **Processing questions for the clients (Preguntas de proceso para los/as clientes)**

1. After reading the microfiction, what is the very first reaction that comes to your mind? Explain. (*Después de leer la microficción, ¿cuál es la primera reacción que te viene a la mente? Explicar.*)

2. Imagine that you are the main character walking the streets of St. Petersburg, Russia. What was lacking in his life prior to making contact with the two men living on the street? Speculate. (*Imagina que eres el personaje principal caminando por las calles de San Petersburgo, Rusia, ¿qué te faltaba en tu vida antes de tener contacto con los dos deambulantes en la calle? Especular.*)

3. What was the definition of daily living for the main character before and after the encounter on the street? Elaborate. (*¿Cuál fue la definición de la vida diaria del protagonista antes y después del encuentro en la calle? Elaborar.*)

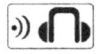 **Sayings (*dichos*)**

 ***Saying #1***

"What more mystery and gratitude than that of a rooster that faithfully wakes me up every morning without my asking."

*"Qué más misterio y agradecimiento que el de un gallo que me levanta fielmente todas las mañanas sin que yo se lo pida."*

Author: Unknown. Popular Hebrew saying (D. Gabai, C. personal communication, December 4, 2020).

**Processing questions for the clients (Preguntas de proceso para los/as clientes)**

1. Obviously the rooster has an internal mechanism that inspires him to crow in the morning in anticipation of the sunrise. What inspires you to perform your daily activities? Discuss. (*Obviamente, el gallo tiene un mecanismo interno que lo inspira a cantar por la mañana en anticipación al amanecer. ¿Qué te inspira a realizar tus actividades diarias? Discutir.*)

2. If you are walking on the hamster wheel and you seem to be in the same position every day, why have you decided to not step out of the hamster wheel? What's impeding your inspiration? Dialogue. (*Si caminas sobre la rueda de hámster y pareces estar en la misma posición todos los días, ¿por qué has decidido no salir de la rueda de hámster? ¿Qué está impidiendo tu inspiración? Diálogo.*)

3. Are your personal inspirations based on other people's needs or yours? What sacrifices are involved in order to capture your own imagination? List. (*¿Tus inspiraciones personales se basan en las necesidades de otras personas o en las tuyas? ¿Qué sacrificios están involucrados para capturar su propia imaginación? Lista.*)

 *Saying #2*

"If the birds sing every day for the mere fact of having a nest, a tree, light and wings; then, sing!"

  "*Si las aves cantan todas los días por el mero hecho de tener un nido, un árbol, luz y alas; entonces, ¡a cantar!*"

Author: Unknown. Popular Latin American saying (B. Mendoza, personal communication, February 13, 2017).

 **Processing questions for the clients (Preguntas de proceso para los/as clientes)**

1. What is the key message of this popular saying? Discuss. (*¿Cuál es el mensaje clave de este dicho popular? Discutir.*)

2. Wake up early and go to an area where there is wildlife. What information can you extract about the fauna, their reaction about a new day, and their activities? What can you say about yourself when comparing their attitude and energy about life with yours? Explain. (*Levántate temprano y diríjete a un área donde haya vida silvestre. ¿Qué información puedes extraer sobre la fauna, su reacción ante un nuevo día y sus actividades? ¿Qué puedes decir de ti mismo al comparar su actitud y energía sobre la vida con la tuya? Explicar.*)

3. What has inspired you to do unique and interesting activities in your life in the past? How long have you kept this inspiration? Cite them and elaborate. (*¿Qué te ha inspirado a realizar actividades únicas e interesantes en tu vida en el pasado? ¿Cuánto tiempo llevas guardando esta inspiración? Cítalos y explícalos.*)

**Quotes**

 *Quote #1*

> "Live as if you were to die tomorrow. Learn as if you were to live forever."
> *"Vive como si fueras a morir mañana. Aprende como si fueras a vivir para siempre."*

Author: Mahatma Gandhi (2021). He was an Indian lawyer, anti-colonial nationalist, and political ethicist who employed nonviolent resistance to lead the successful campaign for India's independence from British rule and in turn inspired movements for civil rights and freedom across the world.

**Processing questions for the clients (Preguntas de proceso para los/as clientes)**

1. What inspirational message can you extract from this quote? Explain. (*¿Qué mensaje inspirador puedes extraer de esta cita? Explicar.*)
2. What has learning taught you about living and inspiration in life? Provide specific examples. (*¿Qué te ha enseñado el aprendizaje sobre la vida y la inspiración en la vida? Proporciona ejemplos específicos.*)
3. If you could change one thing about your life in general, what would it be? And, how can learning help you to find inspiration to pursue something? Dialogue. (*Si pudieras cambiar algo de tu vida en general, ¿qué sería? Y, ¿cómo puede el aprendizaje ayudarte a encontrar inspiración para perseguir algo? Diálogo.*)

*Quote #2*

> "I have not failed. I've just found 10,000 ways that won't work."
> *"No he fallado. Acabo de encontrar 10,000 formas que no funcionarán."*

Author: Thomas A. Edison (Dickson & Dickson, 1894).

**Processing questions for the clients (Preguntas de proceso para los/as clientes)**

1. It is clear that the author of the quote is sending a message of persistence.
2. Can you recall the times that you have failed many times at something and how does this quote re-inspire you to continue? (*Está claro que el autor de la cita está enviando un mensaje de perseverancia.¿Puedes recordar las veces que has fallado muchas veces en algo y cómo esta cita puede volver a inspirarte a continuar?*)
3. Are you typically inspired only by positive emotional waves or negative events? Provide specific illustrations. (*¿Sueles estar inspirado solo por ondas emocionales positivas o eventos negativos? Proporciona ilustraciones específicas.*)
4. **Pledge of Inspiration**. Complete the following Pledge of Inspiration and place it in a location in which you can read it on a daily basis. On the side, have another piece of paper to record the moments in which the inspiration was pursued or quelched. (***Compromiso de inspiración.*** *Complete el siguiente Juramento de inspiración y colócalo en un lugar en el que puedas leerlo a diario. A un lado, ten otra hoja de papel para registrar los momentos en los que te persiguió o apagó la inspiración.*)

*Personal Contract*

I am _____ years old. In the past, I have let other people ridicule my ideas, inspirations, and plans. I declare that today_____, I will seek out something that inspires me to continue on this journey. I am in constant pursuit of the inspiration that allows me to be fulfilled in life. Be it materialistic, spiritual, emotional or physical, I declare ownership over my inspiration and declare it a reality in my life.

Signature_____

*Contrato personal*

*Tengo _____ años. En el pasado, dejé que otras personas ridiculizaran mis ideas, inspiraciones y planes. Declaro que hoy _____, buscaré algo que me inspire a continuar en este camino. Estoy en constante búsqueda de la inspiración que me permita realizarme en la vida. Ya sea materialista, espiritual, emocional o física. Declaro propiedad sobre mi inspiración y la declaro una realidad en mi vida.*

*Firma_____*

 **Quote #3**

"Life isn't about finding yourself. Life is about creating yourself."
*"Nunca es demasiado tarde para ser lo que podrías haber sido."*

Author: George Bernard Shaw (2015). He was an Irish playwright, critic, polemicist, and political activist.

 **Processing questions for the clients (Preguntas de proceso para los/as clientes)**

1. What is the key message from this quote as you see it today? Explain. (*¿Cuál es el mensaje clave de esta cita como la ves hoy? Explicar.*)
2. What is the difference between finding yourself and creating yourself? List differences. (*¿Cuál es la diferencia entre encontrarte a ti mismo y crearte a ti mismo? Enumera las diferencias.*)
3. Do you think that the process of "finding yourself" might be some type of self-fulling prophecy or personally pre-determined strategy to explain the failures in your life and, therefore, remain stuck in life? That is, what if you find yourself and you do not like what you see? Instead, and based on the quote, and through a process of self-empowerment, you might be able to short-circuit this self-defeating process and "create" a new you. See the picture that follows of a human being and make an arrow to the areas in your life that you want to create. This might be literal, spiritual, emotional, psychological, physical, relational, social, career, a specific trait, etc. Once you connect the arrows to the image, explain how this new part of you would look like. (*¿Crees que el proceso de "encontrarte a ti mismo" podría ser algún tipo de profecía autocumplida o una estrategia predeterminada personalmente para explicar los fracasos en tu vida y, por lo tanto, quedarte estancado en la vida? Es decir, ¿y si te encuentras a ti mismo y no te gusta lo que ves? En cambio, y según*

*la cita, y a través de un proceso de auto-empoderamiento, es posible que puedas cortocircuitar este proceso contraproducente y "crear" un nuevo yo. Ve la imagen de abajo de un ser humano y haz una flecha en las áreas de tu vida que deseas crear. Esto puede ser literal, espiritual, emocional, psicológico, físico, relacional, social, profesional, un rasgo específico, etc. Una vez que conectes las flechas con la imagen, explica cómo se vería esta nueva parte de ti.)*

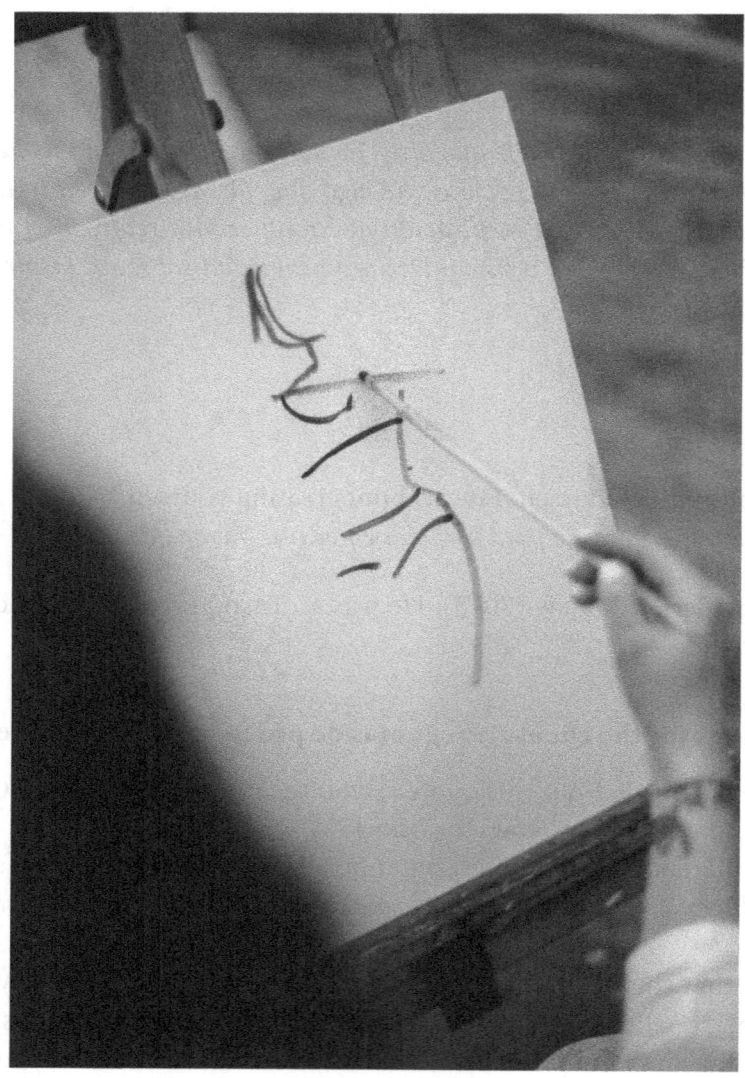

*Figure 18.1* Woman's Hand Sketching a Figure

## References

Dickson, W. K., & Dickson, A. (1894). *The life and inventions of Thomas Alva Edison*. Chatto & Windus.

Gandhi, M. (2021, July 7). www.brainyquote.com/quotes/mahatma_gandhi_133995

Shaw, G. B. (2015). *George Bernard Shaw—An unsocial socialist: "Life isn't about finding yourself. Life is about creating yourself"*. Word to the Wise.

# 19 Motivation

Motivation is a powerful force that can help human beings to chase goals and dreams, surpass pain or a disease, and stay alive. Decreased motivation in some clients inhibits them to reach their full potential and prevents them from succeeding in their life endeavors. Motivation can be found in the more obvious daily experiences as interpreted by each person or it can be suppressed if not sufficiently nurtured. The people who have experienced the most transformational experiences in life attribute it to internal or intrinsic factors that serve as unlimited fuel even during the most difficult times. External motivation can be short-lived especially if it is pushed by someone else. However, if the extrinsic experience can be easily converted into an internal motivation it can last longer and be maintained by internal accountability. This is one of the most powerful goals to be instilled in our clients in order to prevent overdependence on the counselor or extrinsic motivation.

See also: hope, focus, self-realization, change, and future

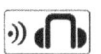 **Microfiction**

### The Morning

It was 5:00 am, and the alarm clock woke me up. Why? Why? A moment of silence. An invasion of thoughts. "Stay in bed, stay in bed, rest, don't leave the warmth of your bed. It's not worth it after all. Just one morning." I remember the desperation of my parents trying to feed each one of my siblings. Necessity, poverty, scarcity. Fear. I woke up. The lights of cars can be seen through my window. I say to myself: "If they woke up and are already on the road, they are no better than me, they are pursuing their dreams. I am already behind! Dream, I am after you, I will chase you today. Today is the day!"

(*Español*)

 **Microficción**

### La Mañana

*Son las 5:00 am, el despertador me despertó. ¿Por qué? ¿Por qué? Un momento de silencio. Una invasión de pensamientos. "Quédate en la cama, quédate en la cama, descansa, no dejes la tibieza*

DOI: 10.4324/9781003145943-23

*de tu cama. Después de todo, no vale la pena. Solo una mañana". Recuerdo la desesperación de mis padres tratando de alimentar a cada uno de mis hermanos. Necesidad, pobreza, escasez. Miedo. Me despierto. Las luces de los autos se pueden ver a través de mi ventana. Me digo a mí mismo: "Si se despertaron y ya están en el camino, no son mejores que yo, están persiguiendo sus sueños. ¡Ya estoy atrasado! Sueño, te persigo, te perseguiré hoy. ¡Hoy es el día!"*

  Author: Roberto Swazo.

 *Cultural Hints*

Wellness is defined differently from culture to culture. In the West, wellness is emphasized by physical health and vigor. In Eastern cultures, wellness implies a deeper spiritual internal balance rather than physical appearance or strength.

 **Processing questions for the clients (Preguntas de proceso para los/as clientes)**

1. Describe the sensations that the person is experiencing. Elaborate. (*Describe las sensaciones que está experimentando la persona. Elabore.*)
2. What role does the past play in this person? Elaborate. (*¿Qué papel juega en esta persona su pasado? Elabore.*)
3. What motivates this person to keep going even if they are tired? (*¿Qué es lo que motiva a esta persona a seguir aunque esté cansado/a?*)
4. And to you, what motivates you in life? (*Y a ti, ¿qué es lo que te motiva en la vida?*)
5. Make a list of the things that prevent you from achieving what you want. (*Haz una lista de las cosas que te impiden alcanzar lo que tu quieres.*)
6. Where do your motivations come from? Are these external or internal? (*¿De dónde se originan sus motivaciones? ¿Estas son externas o internas?*)

 *Cultural Hints*

Motivation to achieve something can be perceived or construed as a dominant Western value. It is a strong intrinsic value based on an Internal Locus of Control. However, some Eastern cultures are also high achievement oriented and this might be completely relevant as well. The difference might be that in some Eastern countries, the personal achievement of one is a reflection of the collective achievement and success of all.

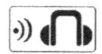 **Sayings (*dichos*)**

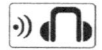 *Saying #1*

  "Better a man who wants and dreams today than the one who complains and regrets tomorrow."
    "*Más vale el hombre que quiere y sueña hoy que el que se queja y lamenta mañana.*"

  Author: Unknown. Popular Latin American saying (A. Llanos, personal communication, February 8, 2017).

**Processing questions for the clients (Preguntas de proceso para los/as clientes)**

1. Make a drawing or a painting that represents what you really want to do. (*Haz un dibujo o una pintura que represente lo que realmente quieres hacer.*)
2. Make another drawing or a painting that represents what you never wanted to do but still do. (*Haz otro dibujo o una pintura que represente lo que nunca has querido hacer pero aun lo sigues haciendo.*)
3. Place both drawings or paintings side by side and describe them. What dreams are possible at this stage of your life? (*Coloque ambos dibujos o pinturas, uno al lado del otro y descríbelos.¿Qué sueños son posibles en esta etapa de tu vida?*)

 *Saying #2*

"Small bull with a big heart opens a huge ditch."
   "*Toro pequeño con corazón grande, abre una zanja inmensa.*"

Author: Unknown. Popular Latin American saying (A. Llanos, personal communication, February 8, 2017).

 **Processing questions for the clients (Preguntas de proceso para los/as clientes)**

1. What do you want in life? (*¿Qué es lo que tu quieres en la vida?*)
2. What are you willing to sacrifice to achieve this? (*¿Qué estás dispuesto/a a sacrificar para alcanzar esto?*)
3. Make a list of the things you anticipate will prevent you from achieving what you want in your life. (*Haz una lista de las cosas que anticipas van a impedir que alcances lo que quieres en tu vida.*)

 **Quotes**

 *Quote #1*

"Necessity, who is the mother of our invention."
   "*Necesidad, aquella que es la madre de nuestra invención.*"

Author: Attributed to Plato and many other folkloric cultures in other forms or versions (Seland, 2017).

 **Processing questions for the clients (Preguntas de proceso para los/as clientes)**

1. What does it mean? (*¿Qué significa la misma?*)
2. Describe what is a necessity for you. (*Describe lo que es una necesidad para ti.*)
3. Make a list of your personal needs. (*Haz una lista de tus necesidades personales.*)
4. From the list, categorize the items between physical, emotional, psychological, economic, spiritual, or other needs. (*De la lista, categoriza la lista entre necesidades físicas, emocionales, psicológicas, económicas, espirituales, u otras.*)

5. Of the previous categories, which one is the most important? Explain. (*De las categorías anteriores, ¿cuál es la más importante? Explique.*)

### *Quote #2*

"I always felt that I hadn't achieved what I wanted to achieve. I always felt I could get better. That's the whole incentive."

  "*Yo siempre sentí que no había logrado lo que quería lograr. Yo siempre sentí que podría hacerlo mejor. Ese era todo mi incentivo.*"

Author: Virginia Wade (Farley & Curry, 1994). She is a former professional tennis player from Great Britain.

### Processing questions for the clients (Preguntas de proceso para los/as clientes)

1. What do you think that you have not achieved in your life? (*¿Qué piensas que nos ha logrado en tú vida?*)
2. What is your reaction to this song? (*¿Cuál es tu reacción a esta canción?*)

   https://www.youtube.com/watch?v=Y66j_BUCBMY (English)
   www.youtube.com/watch?v=VCjUcZrnrHI&list=PLl2gZTdelsIltfrlP1re9m9zuTHHBLrWi (Espanol)

3. Take a big piece of cardboard, place it on the floor, and trace a long thick line from one side to the other. Then, mark points on a continuum of your life in which you have had times of inertia and opportunities have passed by you. Explain. (*Toma un pedazo grande de cartón, colócalo en el piso y traza una línea larga y gruesa de un lado al otro. Luego, marca puntos en un continuo de tu vida en el que hayas tenido momentos de inercia y hayas dejado pasar oportunidades. Explica.*)

### *Quote #3*

"Do not let other people tell you what you want."
  "*No dejes que otras personas te digan lo que usted quiere.*"

Author: Pat Riley (2021). He is an American professional basketball executive and a former coach and player in the National Basketball Association (NBA).

### Processing questions for the clients (Preguntas de proceso para los/as clientes)

1. Describe the picture that follows. (*Describa la foto.*)
2. Describe some moments in your life that you have done things you did not want to do. (*Describe algunos momentos en tu vida que has hecho cosas que no querías hacer.*)
3. Where does your motivation to continue come from? (*¿Dé dónde viene tu motivación para continuar?*)

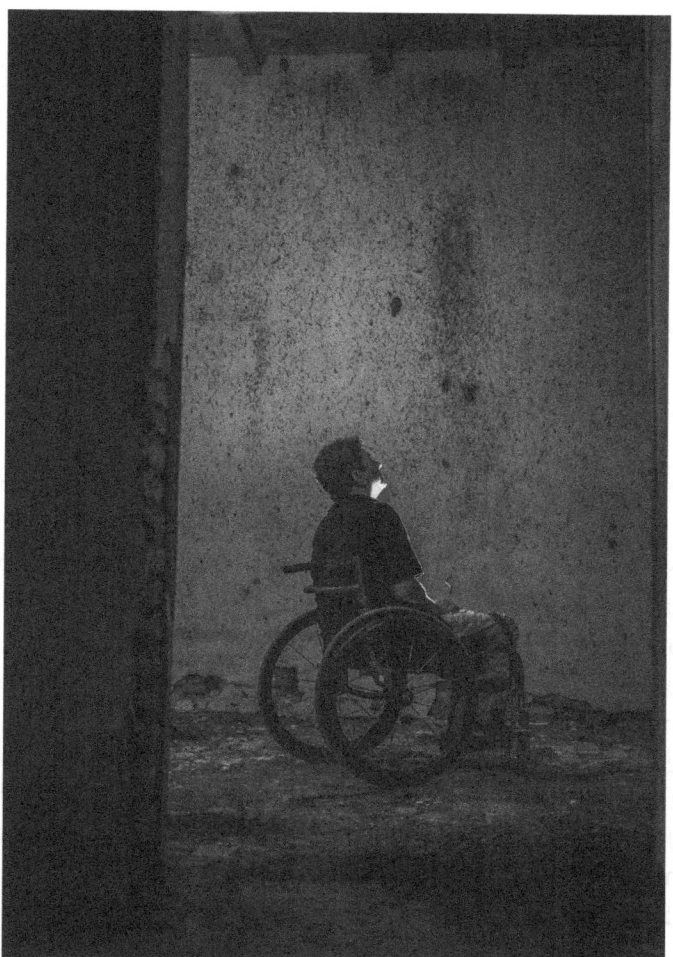

*Figure 19.1* Pensive Person

4.  Take a daily journal and record ALL of your activities, even the most mundane activities, including breaks. Repeat this process for an entire week. Assess your week and determine how much time has been lost, what was purposeful, and where is the motivation to do these coming from? (*Toma un diario y registra TODAS sus actividades, incluso las actividades más mundanas, incluidos los descansos. Repite este proceso durante toda una semana. Evalúa tu semana y determina cuánto tiempo se ha perdido, cuál fue su propósito y de dónde viene la motivación para hacerlo.*)

## References

Farley, K. L., & Curry, S. M. (1994). *Get motivated! Daily psych-ups*. Fireside Book.

Riley, P. (2021, July 7). www.inspiringquotes.us/author/9535-pat-riley

Seland, D. (2017, September). Necessity: The mother of invention . . . sometimes. *Quality, 56*(9), 6. https://link.gale.com/apps/doc/A507814066/AONE?u=anon~d3c0cbc3&sid=googleScholar&xid=a0d29b04

# 20 Self-Realization

Self-realization always starts with a series of questions and reflections that typically commence with a starting point in life where there is some sense of discomfort with where one is within that continuum. These self-evaluation processes lead to additional questions that will eventually clear the path to the realization that there is inner potential and it is within one's choice to reach it. This sense of awareness creates the modification of purpose resulting in life's directionality. This is a quest that derives in personal satisfaction, contentment, inner peace, and the full exploitation of one's talents and gifts. Although it logically sounds like every human being should pursue self-realization, not every individual knows how to peel off the layers of insecurity, social conventions, familial and cultural expectations, and fears of being oneself. Many clients struggle with feelings of unworthiness and dissatisfaction with their own lives knowing intuitively that they have not reached their full potential.

See also: inspiration, future, hope, and peace

 ## Microfiction

### The Rescued Bird

In the outskirts of a big city, right where the boundaries of the green mountains connected to the forest, a flock of pigeons was congregating as usual. A female pigeon with her partner heard the sounds of alarm and pain from a baby bird that was at the base of a very tall tree. With caution, both pigeons approached the base of the tree and noticed the presence of a baby bird that could not fly as it was either abandoned by her parents or had inadvertently fallen off the bird's nest at the top of the tall tree. With great compassion and love, both pigeons decided to rescue the baby bird and bring it to their family's nest with the rest of their baby pigeons. This bird was significantly bigger in spite of not having grown feathers yet, and to the naked eye, she looked like a ball of fur. The rest of the pigeon community made fun of the foster pigeon parents for bringing such an ugly bird to their community. However, the rescued bird was loved by her pigeon parents as well as her siblings. The parents had to do three to four food gathering shifts in order to feed the adopted bird alone. They noticed that the rescued bird did not care about seeds and fruits but had an insatiable appetite for worms and anything that was meat-based. The rescued bird grew to be an enormous specimen and the pigeon parents hid her from the

DOI: 10.4324/9781003145943-24

community in order to protect her from the constant bullying and criticism from the pigeon neighbors. One day, the pigeon community came under attack by a powerful constrictor snake that was wreaking havoc throughout the pigeon community by eating the baby pigeons from their nests as well as some of their protective parents who refused to leave their babies at the mercy of the gigantic snake. Suddenly, like a lightning bolt coming through the dense tree foliage, an immense eagle stabbed her powerful talons into the flesh of the gigantic snake, climbed high in the sky, and slammed it against a nearby cliff to later devour it. In disbelief, the pigeon community realized that this was the adopted bird by their pigeon neighbors. It was not an ugly bird but a beautiful, powerful, and majestic golden eagle flying above the forest like a Greek god protecting the pigeon community.

(Español)

 ## Microficción

### *El Ave Rescatada*

*En las afueras de una gran ciudad, justo donde los límites de las verdes montañas conectaban con la jungla, una bandada de palomas se congregaba como de costumbre. Una paloma hembra con su compañero escuchó los sonidos de alarma y dolor de un pájaro bebé que estaba en la base de un árbol muy alto. Con precaución, ambas palomas se acercaron a la base del árbol y notaron la presencia de un pájaro bebé que no podía volar ya que fue abandonado por sus padres o se había caído inadvertidamente del nido del pájaro en la parte superior del árbol alto. Con gran compasión y amor, ambas palomas decidieron rescatar al pajarito y llevarlo al nido de su familia con el resto de sus palomas bebé. Esta ave era significativamente más grande a pesar de que todavía no le habían crecido las plumas, y a simple vista parecía una bola de pelo. El resto de la comunidad de palomas se burló de los padres adoptivos por traer un pájaro tan feo a su comunidad. Sin embargo, el pájaro rescatado fue amado por sus padres las palomas, así como por sus hermanos. Los padres tuvieron que hacer tres o cuatro turnos de recolección de alimentos para alimentar sólo al ave adoptada. Notaron que al pájaro rescatado no le importaban las semillas y las frutas, pero tenía un apetito insaciable por los gusanos y cualquier cosa que fuera a base de carne. El pájaro rescatado se convirtió en un espécimen enorme y los padres palomas la escondieron de la comunidad para protegerla del constante acoso y las críticas de los vecinos de la comunidad de palomas. Un día, la comunidad de palomas fue atacada por una poderosa serpiente constrictora que estaba causando estragos en toda la comunidad de palomas al comerse a las crías de sus nidos, así como a algunos de sus padres protectores que se negaron a dejar a sus bebés a merced de la gigante serpiente. De repente, como un rayo de luz que atraviesa la densidad del denso follaje de los árboles, un águila inmensa apuñaló sus poderosas garras sobre la carne de la gigantesca serpiente, trepó al cielo y lo golpeó contra un acantilado cercano para luego devorarlo. Con incredulidad, la comunidad de palomas se dio cuenta de que este era el ave adoptada por sus vecinos. No era un pájaro feo, sino un águila real hermosa, poderosa y majestuosa que volaba sobre el bosque como un dios griego que protege a la comunidad de palomas.*

Author: Roberto Swazo.

·)) ◖🎧◗   *Cultural Hints*

Self-realization might be a foreign concept for some in which collective success is more important than personal development. That being said, there is always a continuum of individuality and uniqueness for every individual within a determined culture regardless of the dominant social conventions.

·)) ◖🎧◗   **Processing questions for the clients (Preguntas de proceso para los/as clientes)**

1.  Have you ever felt different and rejected from/by others? Do you feel that those around you value all of your potential? Elaborate. (*¿Alguna vez te has sentido diferente y rechazado del resto de los demás? ¿Sientes que los que te rodean valoran todo tu potencial? Elaborar.*)

2.  Do you think that the adopted eagle held a grudge? How come the golden eagle defended the community of pigeons after being bullied during her infancy and adolescence? Explain. (*¿Crees que el águila adoptada guardaba rencor? ¿Cómo es que el águila real defendió a la comunidad de palomas después de haber sido intimidada durante su infancia y adolescencia? Explique.*)

3.  What has prevented you from expressing your true potential in life? Be specific. (*¿Qué te ha impedido expresar tu verdadero potencial en la vida? Se especí fico.*)

4.  Complete the following incomplete sentences, process the content and elaborate.

    a.  When I was growing up people said that I was _____.
    b.  My parents or caretakers believed that I was _____.
    c.  When I look at the mirror I see a_____.
    d.  I believe that I am _____.

    (*Completa las siguientes oraciones incompletas, procesa el contenido y elabora. Cuando era niño, la gente decía que yo era _____. Mis padres o cuidadores creían que yo era _____. Cuando miro al espejo veo un _____. Creo que soy _____ _____.*)

5.  Complete the sections (fill the blanks) of this *story* and explain:

    Once upon a time there was a kid who _____. At times the kid felt _____. During difficult times the kid behaved as if _____. The kid's life changed when _____. The kid looked for solutions to cope with difficulties by _____. The kid grew up to be an adult but _____ _____.

    [*Complete las secciones (llene los espacios en blanco) de esta historia y explique:*

    *Había una vez un niño que _____. A veces el niño sintió _____. Durante tiempos difíciles, el niño se comportó como si _____. La vida del niño cambió cuando _____. El niño buscó soluciones para hacer frente a las dificultades por _____. El niño creció para ser adulto pero _____.*]

**Sayings (*dichos*)**

 ***Saying #1***

"Give time to time and find yourself in time."
*"Dale tiempo al tiempo y encuéntrate con el tiempo."*

Author: Unknown. Popular Latin American saying (C. Castillo, personal communication, February 9, 2017).

 **Processing questions for the clients (Preguntas de proceso para los/as clientes)**

1. What's the meaning of this quote? Is your current interpretation different from the one that you would have given to it some years ago? What's different? Explain. (*¿Cuál es el significado de esta cita? ¿Es tu interpretación actual diferente de la que le hubieses dado hace algunos años? ¿Qué es diferente? Explica.*)
2. Have you used time effectively to find yourself? What does it mean to find yourself? Elaborate. (*¿Has usado el tiempo efectivamente para encontrarte a ti mismo? ¿Qué significa encontrarte a ti mismo? Elaborar.*)
3. Make a list of the things that have prevented you from finding yourself and the potential that you have? From this list, how many could have been prevented and were under your control? Of these, how many can be changed? How can these be changed? What is the outcome of these changes? (*Hacer una lista de las cosas que te han impedido encontrarte a ti mismo y el potencial que tienes. De esta lista, ¿cuántos podrían haberse evitado y estar bajo su control? De estos, ¿cuántos se pueden cambiar? ¿Cómo se pueden cambiar? ¿Cuál es el resultado de estos cambios?*)

 ***Saying #2***

"Whoever gets up early God helps him, and he who is lost finds himself."
*"El que madruga Dios lo ayuda, y el que está perdido se encuentra."*

Author: Unknown. Popular Latin American saying (M. Aguilar, personal communication, February 16, 2017).

 **Processing questions for the clients (Preguntas de proceso para los/as clientes)**

1. Waking up early is a symbol of specifically, what? Interpret and discuss. (*Despertarse temprano es un simbolismo de específicamente ¿qué? Interpretar y discutir.*)
2. Who is your hero or heroine? What's attractive about them? Do you think that this person found themselves? In what way? Where are you in the journey of finding yourself? (*¿Quién es tu héroe o heroína? ¿Qué es lo atractivo de él o ella? ¿Crees que esta persona se encontró a sí misma? ¿De qué manera? ¿Dónde estás en el viaje de encontrarte a tí mismo?*)
3. Do you have a preferred song that serves as inspiration to you to become all the best you can be? Share it, write it down, play the melody in your head. What's special about it? (*¿Tienes una canción preferida que te sirva de inspiración para convertirte en lo mejor que puedas ser? Compártela, escríbela, toca la melodía en tu cabeza. ¿Qué tiene de especial?*)

## Quotes

### Quote #1

"Buddha was asked: 'What have you gained from meditation?' And, he replied: 'Nothing!' However, Buddha said, 'let me tell you what I lost: anger, anxiety, depression, insecurity, fear of old age, and death.'"

*"Se le preguntó a Buda: '¿Qué has ganado de la meditación?' Y él respondió: '¡Nada!' "Sin embargo, dijo Buda, 'déjame decirte lo que perdí: ira, ansiedad, depresión, inseguridad, miedo a la vejez y muerte'."*

Author: The Buddha (also known as Siddhattha Gotama or Siddhārtha Gautama) was a philosopher, mendicant, meditator, spiritual teacher, and religious leader who lived in ancient India (c. 5th to 4th century BCE). He is the founder of the world religion of Buddhism (Pal, 2016).

### Processing questions for the clients (Preguntas de proceso para los/as clientes)

1. Find a quiet place where no one can interrupt you. Turn off the phone, TV, and stay away from your personal computer. Close your eyes and engage in a breathing exercise, relax all your muscles, and declutter your mind. Now, if you could have a different life, who would you like to be? Describe this person. What activities would you like to do? Who are you with? Where do you live? Are you happy and content? How do you look physically and psychologically? What do you need, in order to be this ideal person? Discuss. (*Encuentra un lugar tranquilo donde nadie pueda interrumpirte. Apaga el teléfono, la televisión y mantente alejado de tu computadora personal. Cierra los ojos y realiza un ejercicio de respiración, relaja todos tus músculos y despeja tu mente. Ahora, si pudieras tener una vida diferente, ¿quién te gustaría ser? Describe a esta persona. ¿Qué actividades te gustaría hacer? ¿Con quién estás? ¿Dónde vives? ¿Estás feliz y contento? ¿Cómo te ves física y psicológicamente? ¿Qué necesitas para ser la persona ideal? Discutir.*)

2. Make a list of people whom you have a relationship with and whom you are comfortable enough to ask questions. Try to set up coffee/tea, lunches, or dinners with them separately. Engage them in a conversation and ask them in a candid way for their honest opinions. Process their answers, and since these are people who are similar to you, then you have to realize if they are truly self-realized, if they are giving you honest answers, or perhaps they are in a self-exploration journey as well. Ask them: (*Haz una lista de las personas con las que tienes una relación y con las que te sientes lo suficientemente cómodo como para hacerles preguntas. Intenta hacer citas de café/té, almuerzos o cenas con ellos por separado. Involúcralos en una conversación y pídeles de manera sincera sus opiniones honestas. Procesa sus respuestas, y dado que se trata de personas que son similares a ti, entonces debes darte cuenta de si son realmente autorrealizadas, si te están dando respuestas honestas, o tal vez también están en un viaje de auto-exploracion. Pregúntales:*)

    a. Do you feel self-realized? When did you realize this? At what point in your life did you reach that conclusion? How are you different now from before when you were not self-realized? (*¿Te sientes autorrealizado? ¿Cuándo te diste cuenta de esto? ¿En qué punto de tu vida llegaste a esa conclusión? ¿En qué te diferencias ahora de antes cuando no estabas autorrealizado?*)

b. What strategies did you use to get to that point? (*¿Qué estrategias usaste para llegar a ese punto?*)

c. How has time changed you? (*¿Cómo te ha cambiado el tiempo?*)

3. Going along with the quote from Budha in which he indicates that he has lost anger, anxiety, depression, insecurity, fear of old age, and death through meditation, take time to watch the video *Taoism: The Power of Letting Go. www.youtube.com/watch?v=B-F319b5SuQ* (*Siguiendo la cita de Buda en la que indica que ha perdido la ira, la ansiedad, la depresión, la inseguridad, el miedo a la vejez y la muerte a través de la meditación, tómese el tiempo para ver el video El Arte de Cerrar Ciclos:*

*www.youtube.com/watch?v=PgWl93IbPuU*)

a. Identify with a degree of specificity all the things that you have to let go that are meaningless and do not add any value to your life. (*Identifique con un grado de especificidad todas las cosas que tiene que dejar ir que no tienen sentido y no agregan ningún valor a su vida.*)

b. From the previous list, how many of these are emotional and psychological in nature? And, how many of these are material or physical? What does it say about your current life? (*De la lista anterior, ¿cuántos de estos son de naturaleza emocional y psicológica? Y, ¿cuántos de estos son materiales o físicos? ¿Qué dice sobre tu vida actual?*)

c. Create a plan of simplistic reductionism and week by week start eliminating elements from this week. Evaluate yourself monthly. Be honest with yourself. If you find yourself returning to previous behaviors that were negatively repetitive with destructive patterns, make efforts to reassess and find new strategies to eliminate this. The ultimate goal is to self-realize and unleash all your personal potential. (*Crea un plan de reduccionismo simplista y semana a semana comienza a eliminar elementos de esa semana. Evalúate mensualmente. Sé honesto contigo mismo. Si encuentras regresiones a comportamientos previos que fueron negativamente repetitivos con patrones destructivos, haz esfuerzos para reevaluar y encontrar nuevas estrategias para eliminar esto. El objetivo final es autorrealizarse y liberar todo tu potencial personal.*)

 *Quote #2*

"Radical acts of self-transformation do not occur spontaneously, meaningful change requires a specific and deliberative act of will."

"*Los actos radicales de autotransformación no ocurren espontáneamente, un cambio significativo requiere un acto de voluntad específico y deliberativo.*"

Author: Kilroy J. Oldster is an accomplished trial attorney, arbitrator, and mediator and author of the *Dead Toad Scrolls* (2015).

**Processing questions for the clients (Preguntas de proceso para los/as clientes)**

1. According to the quote, in order to achieve radical self-transformation one has to be deliberate about it. What does this mean specifically in your life? Explain. (*Según la cita, para lograr una auto transformación radical, uno debe ser deliberado al respecto. ¿Qué significa esto específicamente en tu vida? Explique.*)

2. Are you a believer in destiny? If so, do you believe that events in your life have been predestined and you have limited influence in their outcome? (*¿Eres un creyente en el destino? Si es así, ¿crees que los eventos en tu vida han sido predestinados y tienen una influencia limitada en su resultado?*)

3. What is your immediate and unfiltered reaction when you see the following pictures of people? Do you feel admiration or envy? Do you immediately label them as filthy rich and loaded? Do you say to yourself that they are wealthy but unhappy? Discuss. (*¿Cuál es su reacción inmediata y sin filtro cuando ve imágenes de las personas a continuación? ¿Sientes admiración o envidia? ¿Los etiquetas inmediatamente como asquerosamente ricos y cargados? ¿Te dices a ti mismo que son ricos pero infelices? Discute.*)

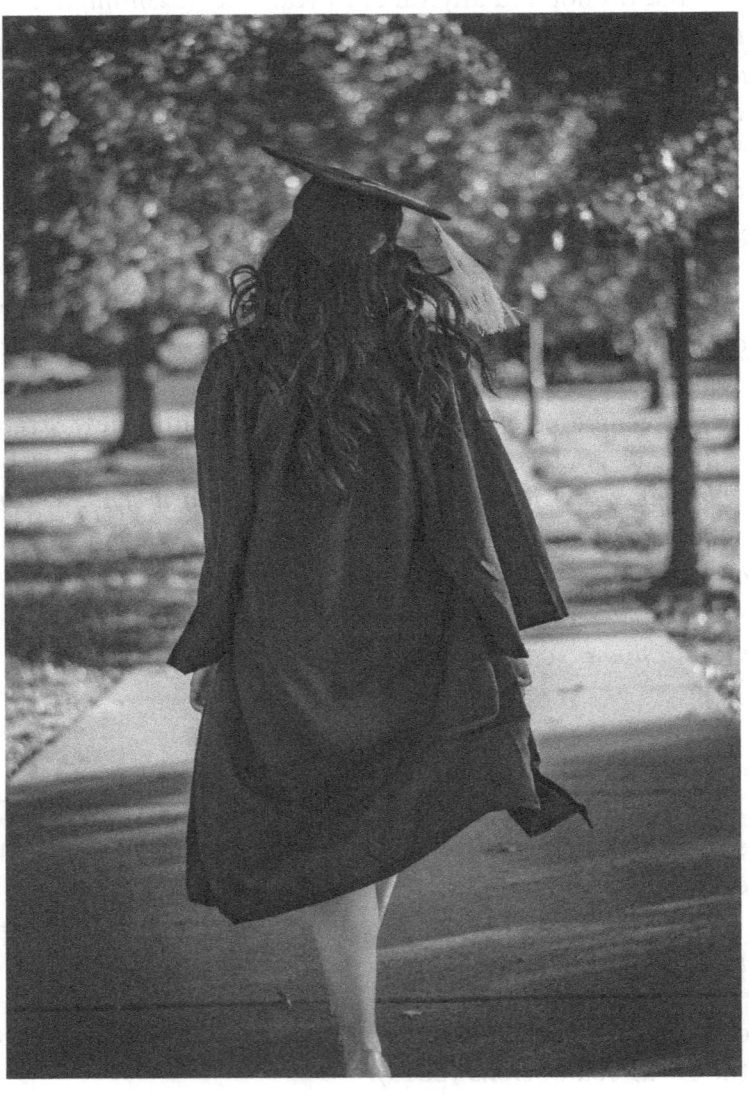

*Figure 20.1*  Recent Graduate

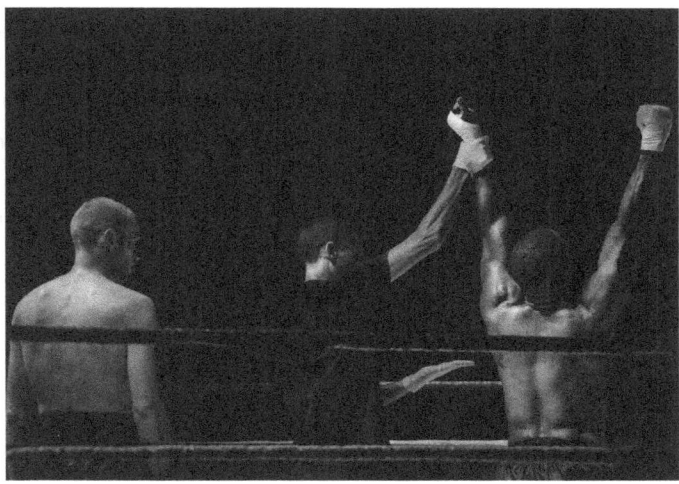

*Figure 20.2* Boxer With Arm Raised in Victory

### Quote #3

"Never compete with others, you are not running the same race."
   *"Nunca compitas con otros, no estás corriendo la misma carrera."*

Author: Gift Gugu Mona is a South African born poet, philosopher, songwriter, and a philanthropist (2021). She is a doctor in public health and advocates for the transformation of lives.

### Processing questions for the clients (Preguntas de proceso para los/as clientes)

1. Break down the preceding quote and determine what it means to you today. Elaborate. (*Desglosa la cita anterior y determina lo que significa hoy para ti. Elaborar.*)
2. Based on the picture that follows, who have you been competing with in your life? That includes family, siblings, friends, school, college, coworkers, etc. Explain and provide examples. (*Según la imagen a continuación, ¿contra quién has estado corriendo en tu vida? Esto incluye familia, hermanos, amigos, escuela, universidad, compañeros de trabajo, etc. Explica y brinda ejemplos.*)

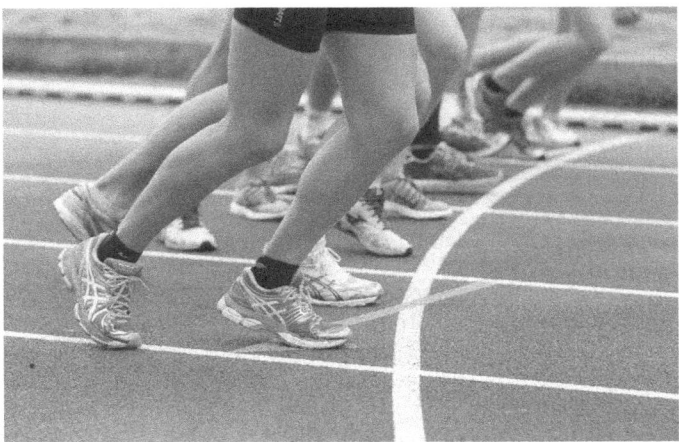

*Figure 20.3* Individuals Racing

3. Do you believe that self-realization is achieved when you have competed against someone, a societal standard, or an imposed cultural standard? Provide your definition of self-realization. Discuss. (*¿Crees que la autorrealización se logra cuando compites contra alguien, un estándar social o un estándar cultural impuesto? Proporciona tu definición de autorrealización. Discutir.*)

4. Make a list of the areas of your life that you feel remain undeveloped or unself-realized. From the list, which are self-imposed expectations and which are criteria imposed by others? How do you differentiate success from self-realization? Elaborate. (*Haz una lista de las áreas de tu vida que sientes que no están desarrolladas o que no se han realizado. De la lista, cuáles son expectativas autoimpuestas y cuáles son criterios impuestos por otros. ¿Cómo diferenciar el éxito de la autorrealización? Elaborar.*)

## References

Mona, G. G. (2021, May 27). www.goodreads.com/quotes/9292685-never-compete-with-others-you-are-not-running-the-same

Oldster, K. J. (2015). *Dead toad scrolls*. Booklocker.com, Incorporated.

Pal, R. (2016). *A treasury of wisdom*. Partridge Publishing India.

# 21 Hope

Hope is one of the principal pillars for human survival under extreme conditions. Hope is one of those core beliefs that surpass logic or reasoning and provide the extra drive force to surpass what appears to be a series of insurmountable obstacles. Unlike a dream or a flight of fancy in which "wishes" are seen as a mirage in the horizon, hope carries a heavier force anchored in more than wishful thinking but an internal fire that lights the way to a new reality. It is contested by existential therapists that without hope humans fall into a state of psychological and emotional decadence that leads to an unfulfilling lifestyle. Hope has many shapes and forms and is executed differently by individuals. But in essence, to give up all hope is the first precondition for any thoughtful effort to overcome the challenges which life sets before us. Hope reveals itself as the solid foundation in which the life of a person is grounded, upholding the individual and preventing them from embarking into nothingness. Hope is the expression of the confidence we set in life and it is accompanied by a sense of gratitude and expectation.

See also: future, change, inspiration, and forgiveness

 **Microfiction**

### Carrying Hope on the Back

The road is steep and muddy, especially after the typical downpour in the mountainous climate of Central America. At a distance, it seems like little multicolor sacks are moving slowly around the mountain towards the main road. In reality, one is unable to see the people that are serving as human mules to carry heavy sacks of grains, fruits, and textiles on their backs. Among them, there is a little girl carrying a sack that almost doubles her in weight and size. Aurora is a 12-year-old native Maya girl who everyday (including weekends) heads up to the main road to catch a public bus (chicken bus) around 5:00 am in order to find a nice spot in town to sell her goods. Conspicuously, she carries a couple of books within the fruits and vegetables. She was taught to read at 7 and dropped out of school at 9 in order to help the family make ends meet. She has five siblings younger than her and she must contribute to the family. One day, while she attended rural school, another native Maya teacher told Aurora that if she studied and got good grades, she could qualify to get a scholarship in the city and be a teacher like her. Then, she would not need to carry heavy sacks

DOI: 10.4324/9781003145943-25

of produce in order to help the family. Moreover, she could even go out of the country and see other people, learn other languages, and explore the world. An old wrinkled and stained geography booklet was all she had to keep the hope alive; she would devour its contents every day and do calculations in order to keep her mathematical abilities sharp. Every day, she would wake up happy and full of energy saying: "Today, I will sell a lot of fruits in the market, save a little for myself and one day will go to the city to test out and finish school, I know it, it's a beautiful day!"

 *Cultural Hints*

Like anything else, hope might be defined differently by everyone. And, an ultimate goal based on hope might seem meaningless to individuals of wealthy nations while it can be an extraordinary accomplishment by others from low SES sectors or poor nations. To clients who have been socially, racially, legally, religiously, and economically oppressed, hope might be interpreted as a privileged concept especially when basic necessities such as food and safety are absent.

(Español)

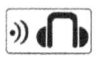 **Microficción**

### *Cargando la Esperanza en la Espalda*

*El camino es empinado y lodoso, especialmente después del típico aguacero en el clima montañoso de Centroamérica. A la distancia, parece que pequeños sacos multicolores se mueven lentamente alrededor de la montaña hacia la carretera principal. En realidad, uno no puede ver a las personas que están sirviendo como mulas humanas para llevar pesados sacos de granos, frutas y textiles en sus espaldas. Entre ellos, hay una niña que lleva un saco que casi le dobla en peso y tamaño. Aurora es una niña maya nativa de 12 años que todos los días (incluidos los fines de semana) se dirige a la carretera principal para tomar un autobús público (autobús de carga de pollos y animales mezclado con personas) alrededor de las 5:00 am para encontrar un lugar agradable en la ciudad para vender sus productos. Llamativamente, lleva un par de libros sobre frutas y verduras. Le enseñaron a leer a los 7 años y abandonó la escuela a los 9 para ayudar a la familia a llegar a fin de mes. Tiene cinco hermanos menores que ella y debe contribuir a la familia. Un día, mientras asistía a una escuela rural, otra maestra maya nativa le dijo a Aurora que si estudiaba y sacaba buenas notas, podría calificar para obtener una beca en la ciudad y ser maestra como ella. Entonces, no necesitaría cargar pesados sacos de productos para ayudar a la familia. Además, incluso podría salir del país y ver a otras personas, aprender otros idiomas y explorar el mundo. Un viejo cuadernillo de geografía arrugado y manchado era todo lo que tenía para mantener viva la esperanza, devoraría su contenido todos los días y haría cálculos para mantener afiladas sus habilidades matemáticas. Todos los días se despertaba feliz y llena de energía diciendo: "hoy voy a vender muchas frutas en el mercado, me ahorraré un poco y un día iré a la ciudad a hacer las pruebas y terminar la escuela, lo sé, ¡es un hermoso día!"*
Author: Roberto Swazo.

**Processing questions for the clients (Preguntas de proceso para los/as clientes)**

1. What is your first impression when you read this short story? Discuss. (*¿Cuál es tu primera impresión cuando lees este cuento? Discutir.*)
2. Aurora has a strong drive and high levels of hope in spite of her oppressive situation; can you get into her mind and determine the factors that are driving her forward? List them. (*Aurora tiene un fuerte impulso y altos niveles de esperanza a pesar de su opresiva situación; ¿Puedes penetrar en su mente y determinar los factores que la impulsan a seguir adelante? Ponlos en una lista.*)
3. How does her attitude and hope levels compare to yours and what is currently lacking in order to identify elements that bring about hope in your life? Elaborate. (*¿Cómo se compara su actitud (Aurora) y sus niveles de esperanza con los tuyos y qué te falta actualmente para identificar los elementos que generan esperanza en tu vida? Elaborar.*)
4. What are you currently carrying on your back? Are you carrying unnecessary weight that is dragging you down or feeding your hope? (*¿Qué llevas en la espalda actualmente? ¿Estás cargando un peso innecesario que te está arrastrando hacia abajo o alimentando tu esperanza?*)

 **Sayings (*dichos*)**

 *Saying #1*

"Hope is the bread of the poor."
   "*La esperanza es el pan de los pobres.*"

Author: Unknown. Popular Latin American saying (Beyssade et al., 2012).

**Processing questions for the clients (Preguntas de proceso para los/as clientes)**

1. What does this saying say about despair? Explain. (*¿Qué dice este dicho sobre la desesperación? Explicar.*)
2. Have you been in a situation in which you have lost a lot and there are limited things to hang onto? What are some things that you have lost and seemingly are irreplaceable? (*¿Has estado en una situación en la que has perdido mucho y hay cosas limitadas a las que aferrarte? ¿Cuáles son algunas de las cosas que has perdido y aparentemente son insustituibles?*)
3. If hope could be "quantifiable," how has hope changed on a scale from 1 to 10 during moments of personal crisis for you? Circle the numbers that represent it and explain this process. [*Si la esperanza pudiera ser "cuantificable", ¿cómo ha cambiado la esperanza en una escala del 1 al 10 durante los momentos de crisis personal para ti? Encierra en un círculo los números que lo representan y explica este proceso.*]

 *Saying #2ab*

2a. "Hope is the last thing you lose."

"*La esperanza es lo último que se pierde.*" (I. Flores, personal communication, February 12, 2017)

2b. "While life lasts, hope is not lost."

"*Mientras dura la vida, la esperanza no está perdida.*" (C. Castillo, personal communication, February 9, 2017)

Authors: Unknown. Popular Latin American sayings.

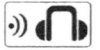 **Processing questions for the clients (Preguntas de proceso para los/as clientes)**

1. Based on both the preceding sayings (2a and b), if you lose everything, how does hope influence one's life? (*Según los dos dichos anteriores (2.a.b), si pierdes todo, ¿cómo influye la esperanza en la vida?*)

2. Select a piece of visual art (i.e., drawing, painting, sculpture) that represents hope to you. If you don't know of one in particular, conduct an Internet research and look for one that represents hope. Have a copy of this and place it by your work area, bedroom, or favorite place in your house. Keep it as an inspiration and emotional reserve for future tough times! (*Selecciona una obra de arte visual (es decir, dibujo, pintura, escultura) que representa esperanza para ti. Si no conoces a nadie en particular, realiza una investigación en Internet y busca uno que represente esperanza. Ten una copia de esto y colócalo junto a tu área de trabajo, dormitorio o lugar favorito de tu casa. ¡Guárdalo como inspiración y reserva emocional para futuros tiempos difíciles!*)

3. Find a quiet place at home, dim the lights, relax, breathe in and out slowly, rid your mind of intrusive thoughts, and center yourself. Once you acquire the desire state of mind, play the following link: (*Encuentra un lugar tranquilo en casa, atenúa las luces, relájate, inhala y exhala lentamente, libera tu mente de pensamientos intrusivos y céntrate. Una vez que adquieras el estado anímico de deseo, reproduce el siguiente enlace:*) Music for Hope and Determination—The Power of One (*Música para la esperanza y la determinación: El poder de uno*)

   https://youtu.be/Olqbdyx9bRQ

Describe your emotions and identify that element, person, higher being, institution, event, etc. that inspires you to generate a wealth of hope. What is it? How can you keep this in your frontal lobe, so to speak? Discuss.

(*Describe tus emociones e identifica ese elemento, persona, ser superior, institución, evento, etc. que te inspira a generar una riqueza de esperanza. ¿Qué es? ¿Cómo puedes mantener esto en tu lóbulo frontal, por así decirlo? Discutir.*)

## Quotes

*Quote #1*

"There is no worse punishment on earth than a fruitless and hopeless task."
"*No hay peor castigo en la tierra que una tarea infructuosa y desesperanzada.*"

Author: Albert Camus (2018). He was a French philosopher, author, and journalist. He won the Nobel Prize in Literature at the age of 44 in 1957. He was the second-youngest recipient in history.

**Processing questions for the clients (Preguntas de proceso para los/as clientes)**

1. Break down this quote. What is the initial thought that comes to your mind? Elaborate. (*Desglosa esta cita, ¿cuál es el pensamiento inicial que te viene a la mente? Elaborar.*)

2. Looking back, have you had days, weeks, months, or years in which the tasks and activities completed lack meaning and you were operating without hope? Describe. (*Mirando hacia atrás, ¿has tenido días, semanas, meses o años en los que las tareas y actividades completadas carecen de significado y has estado operando sin esperanza? Describir.*)

3. If a fruitless and hopeless task is a punishment, then what is the opposite of it? Once you identify (from question 2) those tasks and activities that have been meaningless and hopeless in your life, write down how these can be converted into activities full of hope and meaning. That is, you are preventing repetitive patterns in your life. (*Si una tarea infructuosa y sin esperanza es un castigo, ¿qué es lo opuesto? Una vez que identifiques (de la pregunta 2) aquellas tareas y actividades que no han tenido sentido y han sido desesperadas en tu vida, escribe cómo se pueden convertir en actividades llenas de esperanza y significado. Es decir, estás evitando patrones repetitivos en tu vida.*)

 *Quote #2*

"I am prepared for the worst, but I hope for the best."
"*Estoy preparado para lo peor, pero espero lo mejor.*"

Author: Benjamin Disraeli (in O'Brien, 2015). He was a British politician of Jewish descent and a member of the Conservative Party who twice served as Prime Minister of the United Kingdom.

**Processing questions for the clients (Preguntas de proceso para los/as clientes)**

1. What does the author try to say to you today? Explain. (*¿Qué intenta decirte el autor hoy? Explicar.*)

2. Read the following and respond accordingly (Yes, No, Most of the Time, Rarely). Provide representative examples. (*Lee lo siguiente a continuación y responde en consecuencia (Sí, No, la mayoría de las veces, raras veces). Proporciona ejemplos representativos.*)

   a. ___ I can figure out many creative ways to get out of a difficult situation. (___ *Puedo encontrar muchas formas creativas de salir de una situación difícil.*)

   b. ___ I pursue all my goals with lots of energy, enthusiasm, and determination. (___ *Persigo todas mis metas con mucha energía, entusiasmo y determinación.*)

   c. ___ I can think of many ways to get the things in life that are important to me. (___ *Puedo pensar en muchas formas de conseguir las cosas de la vida que son importantes para mí.*)

   d. ___ Even when my family, friends, and co-workers get dispirited, I remain confident that I can find a way to disentangle the challenges in front of me. (___ *Incluso cuando mi familia, amigos y compañeros de trabajo se desaniman, sigo confiando en que puedo encontrar una manera de desenredar los desafíos que tengo por delante.*)

e.  ___ All my past experiences (negative and positive) have allowed me to be prepared to deal with future situations. (___ *Todas mis experiencias pasadas (negativas y positivas) me han permitido estar preparado para enfrentar situaciones futuras.*)

f.  ___ I always find a way to meet the goals that I set for myself every year. (___ *Siempre encuentro la manera de cumplir con las metas que me propongo cada año.*)

3.  Preparing contingency plans is a contradiction for hope. What do you think? (*¿El preparar planes de contingencia es una contradicción para la esperanza? ¿Qué piensas?*)

## Quote #3

"If I knew that the world would end tomorrow, I, still today, would plant a tree."
"*Si supiera que el mundo se acaba mañana, yo, hoy todavía, plantaría un árbol.*"

Author: Dr. Martin Luther King Jr. (2021). He was an American Christian minister and activist who became the critical catalyst of the civil rights movement from 1955 until his assassination in 1968.

## Processing questions for the clients (Preguntas de proceso para los/as clientes)

1.  What is the key message that the author is trying to communicate? Interpret it. (*¿Cuál es el mensaje clave que el autor está tratando de comunicar? Interprétalo.*)

2.  Based on the following types of hope, which one describes the ones that you have put in action before? (*Basado en los siguientes tipos de esperanza, ¿cuál describe los que has puesto en acción antes?*)

Table 21.1 Dimensions of Hope and Outcomes

| Realistic hope (Esperanza realista) | Realistic hope is hope for an outcome that is reasonable or probable. Being realistic is a way of hoping that allows individuals to observe and understand their situation while still maintaining openness toward the possibility of positive change.<br><br>(*La esperanza realista es la esperanza de un resultado que sea razonable o probable. Ser realista es una forma de esperanza que permite a las personas observar y comprender su situación sin dejar de estar abiertos a la posibilidad de un cambio positivo.*) | Comments (*comentarios*): |
| --- | --- | --- |

| | | |
|---|---|---|
| *Utopian hope* (*Esperanza utópica*) | Is a collectively oriented hope that collaborative action can lead to a better future for all. The utopian hoper critically negates the present and is driven by hope to affirm a better alternative. Consider utopian hope presented by a political movement; a movement that effectively articulates the hopes of a social group to expand the horizons of possibility.<br><br>(*Es una esperanza de orientación colectiva de que la acción colaborativa puede conducir a un futuro mejor para todos. La tolva utópica niega críticamente el presente y está impulsada por la esperanza de afirmar una alternativa mejor. Considera la esperanza utópica presentada por un movimiento político; un movimiento que articula efectivamente las esperanzas de un grupo social para expandir los horizontes de posibilidad.*) | Comments (*comentarios*): |
| *Chosen hope* (*Esperanza elegida*) | Hope not only helps us live with a difficult present but also with an uncertain future. For instance, chosen hope is critical to the management of despair and its accompanying paralysis of action.<br><br>(*La esperanza no solo nos ayuda a vivir con un presente difícil sino también con un futuro incierto. Por ejemplo, la esperanza elegida es fundamental para el manejo de la desesperación y la parálisis de acción que la acompaña.*) | Comments (*comentarios*): |
| *Transcendent hope* (*Esperanza trascendente*)<br><br>1. *Patient hope*—a hope that everything will work out well in the end.<br><br>(*Esperanza paciente: la esperanza de que todo salga bien al final.*) | | Comments (*comentarios*): |

(*Continued*)

*Table 21.1* (Continued)

| | | |
|---|---|---|
| 2. *Generalized hope*—hope not directed toward a specific outcome. (*Esperanza generalizada: esperanza no dirigida hacia un resultado específico.*) | | |
| 3. *Universal hope*—a general belief in the future and a defense against despair in the face of challenges. (*Esperanza universal: una creencia general en el futuro y una defensa contra la desesperación frente a los desafíos.*) | | |

## References

Beyssade, C., Mari, A., & Prete, F. D. (Eds.). (2012). *Genericity*. Oxford University Press.

Camus, A. (2018). *The myth of Sisyphus*. Knopf Doubleday Publishing Group.

King, M, L. (2021, July 7). www.goodreads.com/quotes/35396-even-if-i-knew-that-tomorrow-the-world-would-go

O'Brien, J. K. (2015). *Visions 2100: Stories from your future*. Vivid Publishing.

# 22 Peace

One of the most sought out and yet difficult attributes to incorporate in one's life is the element of peace. The opposite of peace is conflict, chaos, acrimony, and discord. And, chaos is manifested by the lack of harmony and balance. Peace is achieved internally and manifested externally in one's behavior and actions. From a macro social standpoint, peace and balance are elements that many societies crave and have lacked through consistent manifestations of internal and external conflicts. In modern society, human beings pay to go to quiet places such as beaches, mountains, lakes, and country sides with the intent to bring in internal peace to their lives. Peace can be a journey or a destination to many clients from all cultures.

Also see: forgiveness, trust, hope, self-realization, and patience

 ## Microfiction

### *The Squirrel*

The squirrel had been working tirelessly the entire spring, summer, and fall. She was always searching for nuts, seeds, and any other source of food available within the area. She was working from sunrise to sundown, non-stop without taking breaks during the day. She was exhausted and constantly preoccupied about the next winter. Additionally, she wanted to show the rest of the squirrels that she had accumulated more seed wealth than the rest, showing off to demonstrate that she was wealthier than anyone in the forest was one of her goals. She was constantly tormented by her inner soul. Her little head was bombarded by unwanted thoughts, all the time, non-stop. "What if the winter lasts more than normal? What if somebody knows where my supplies are hidden and steals them? What if my seeds are rotted by humidity? What if insects eat away my food supplies? What if there is a forest fire and all my food is burned off? What if, what if . . .?" Tormented, she isolated herself, did not trust anyone, and lived a miserable hermit-like life. Distrustful, full of disdain, and anxiety, her little heart could not take it anymore. There were times that she was out of breath at night, drenched in sweat, agitated, and tormented by all kinds of nightmarish scenarios that were out of her control. After futile attempts to get a hold of her by a neighbor squirrel, some concerned ground squirrels decided to knock on her tree door. To their dismay they found the anxious and conflicted and lonely squirrel dead in the midst of piles and piles of food and supplies.

*(Español)*

DOI: 10.4324/9781003145943-26

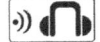

## Microficción

### *La Ardilla*

*La ardilla había estado trabajando incansablemente durante toda la primavera, el verano y el otoño. Ella siempre estaba buscando nueces, semillas y cualquier otra fuente de alimento disponible dentro del área. Ella trabajaba desde el amanecer hasta la puesta del sol, sin parar, sin tomar descansos durante el día. Estaba exhausta y constantemente preocupada por el próximo invierno. Además, quería mostrarle al resto de las ardillas que había acumulado más riqueza de semillas que el resto de las demás. Presumir, demostrar que ella era más rica que nadie en el bosque, ese era uno de sus objetivos. La atormentaba constantemente su alma interior. Su cabecita estaba bombardeada por pensamientos no deseados, todo el tiempo, sin parar. ¿Y si el invierno dura más de lo normal? ¿Qué pasa si alguien sabe dónde están escondidos mis suministros y los roba? ¿Qué pasa si mis semillas se pudren por la humedad? ¿Qué pasa si los insectos se comen mis alimentos? ¿Qué pasa si hay un incendio forestal y toda mi comida se quema? ¿Qué pasa si, qué pasa si . . . ? Atormentada, se aisló, no confiaba en nadie y vivió una vida miserable como ermitaño. Desconfiada, llena de desdén y ansiedad, su pequeño corazón no pudo soportarlo más. Hubo momentos en que estaba sin aliento por la noche, empapada en sudor, agitada y atormentada por todo tipo de escenarios de pesadillas que estaban fuera de control. Después de intentos inútiles de contactarse con ella por una ardilla vecina, algunas ardillas preocupadas decidieron tocar la puerta de su árbol. Para su consternación, encontraron a la ansiosa ardilla, conflictiva y solitaria muerta en medio de montones y montones de alimentos y suministros.*

Author: Roberto Swazo.

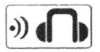

### Processing questions for the clients (Preguntas de proceso para los/as clientes)

1. Based on your initial reaction, what are the main issues faced by the squirrel? Discuss. (*Según tu reacción inicial, ¿cuáles son los principales problemas que enfrenta la ardilla? Discutir.*)

2. It is clear that there are things that can be controlled in our lives and others that cannot be controlled. Make a list of things that you can control, and those that cannot be controlled. Explain. (*Está claro que hay cosas que se pueden controlar en nuestras vidas y otras que no se pueden controlar. Haz una lista de las cosas que puedes controlar y las que no se pueden controlar. Explicar.*)

3. Describe your physical reactions when you experience internal conflicts. Provide details. (*Describe tus reacciones físicas cuando experimentas conflictos internos. Proporcionar detalles.*)

4. Draw concentric circles and rank what occupies the center of your life based on most important (in the most inner circle) to what is least important (outer circle). Feel free to add more concentric circles. Take a closer look at the image, meditate on it. How would you feel if this order were disrupted? What if some of these items were removed and substituted by others? Discuss. (*Dibuja círculos concéntricos, clasifica lo que ocupa el centro de tu vida según su importancia (en el círculo más interno) a lo que es menos importante*

*(círculo externo). Siéntete libre de agregar más círculos concéntricos. Mira más de cerca el imagen, medita en ella. ¿Cómo te sentirías si el orden de las imágenes fueran interrumpidos? ¿Qué pasaría si algunos de estos elementos fueran eliminados y sustituidos por otros? Discutir.)*

 **Sayings (*dichos*)**

 *Saying #1*

> "Better a calm heart than wealth and tormented body."
> *"Mejor corazón tranquilo que riqueza y cuerpo atormentado."*

Author: Unknown. Popular Latin American saying (C. Castillo, personal communication, February 9, 2017).

 **Processing questions for the clients (Preguntas de proceso para los/as clientes)**

1. Attempt to interpret the meaning of this quote. How do you define wealth? (*Interpreta el significado de esta cita. ¿Cómo defines riqueza?*)
2. If you had to choose between being wealthy but tormented by pressure, insecurity, and volatile anxiety versus having a common life but with a limited income, which one would you choose? Explain. (*Si tuvieras que elegir entre ser rico pero atormentado por la presión, la inseguridad y la ansiedad volátil versus tener una vida común pero con un ingreso limitado, ¿cuál elegirías? Explica.*)
3. Try to identify those things that have been cluttering your mind lately. What is important and what's not? Write a list of these cluttering elements, then start writing each one of them on separate pieces of paper. Cross off each one separately, read it out loud, and throw out each one in the basket. Erase them physically and mentally. Experience the calmness of mental decluttering. (*Intenta identificar esas cosas que han estado abarrotando tu mente últimamente. ¿Qué es importante y qué no lo es? Escribe una lista de estos elementos desorganizados, luego, comienza a escribir cada uno de estos por separado en una hoja de papel. Tacha cada uno por separado, léelo en voz alta y tira cada uno en la canasta de basura. Bórralos física y mentalmente. Experimenta la calma de eliminar el destaponamiento/ desorden mental.*)

 *Saying #2*

> "Do not get frustrated by the olives that are out of reach in the high branches but enjoy all the ones that are within your reach."
> *"No te frustres por las aceitunas que están fuera del alcance en las ramas altas, pero disfruta de todas las que están a tu alcance."*

Author: Unknown. Popular Spanish saying (D. Pereira, personal communication, June 12, 2017).

**Processing questions for the clients (Preguntas de proceso para los/as clientes)**

1. Go for a walk on a sunny day. Locate a tree that has some sort of fruit out of reach. Without using a stick to bring it down or climbing up the tree, try to reach as high as possible to get the fruit. Meanwhile, look at all those that are at your reach. What's the meaning and what can be enjoyed now by you? What is out of reach in your life and what is reachable and enjoyable right now? Make a list. (*Sal a caminar en un día soleado. Busca un árbol que tenga algún tipo de fruto fuera de tu alcance. Sin usar un palo para derribarlo o trepar por el árbol, trata de llegar lo más alto posible para obtener la fruta. Mientras tanto, mira todos los que están a tu alcance. ¿Cuál es el significado de esto y que puede ser disfrutado por ti ahora? ¿Qué está fuera del alcance en tu vida y qué es accesible y agradable en este momento? Haz una lista.*)

2. Take some time to reflect every couple of months on whether you're satisfied with the quality of your life. Do you like your current job? Your relationship/s? Based on your current goals and dreams, are you on the right track or are you going through the motions? What adjustments do you have to make in order to restore your inner peace and balance? Discuss. (*Toma un tiempo para reflexionar cada par de meses para ver si estás satisfecho con la calidad de tu vida. ¿Te gusta tu trabajo actual? ¿Tus relación/es? En base a tus metas y sueños actuales, ¿estás en el camino correcto o estás haciendo las cosas de forma automática? ¿Qué ajustes tienes que hacer para restaurar tu paz y equilibrio interior? Discute.*)

## Quotes

 *Quote #1*

"Peace is not the absence of war, it is a virtue, a state of mind, a disposition to benevolence, trust and justice."

"*La paz no es la ausencia de guerra, es una virtud, un estado de la mente, una disposición a la benevolencia, la confianza y la justicia.*"

Author: Baruch Spinoza (2021), Dutch Jewish philosopher, one of the foremost exponents of 17th-century Rationalism and one of the early and seminal figures of the Enlightenment.

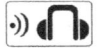 **Processing questions for the clients (Preguntas de proceso para los/as clientes)**

1. If peace is a state of mind, how do you achieve it? What does it look like in your life? If it is a virtue, can you identify it in other people? Make a list of people who seem to have achieved peace with themselves and the world around them. Get together with them, "pick their brains," and ask them for their personal tools to achieve it. Avoid being surrounded by negative individuals whose responses may hinder your progress. (*Si la paz es un estado mental, ¿cómo se logra? ¿Cómo se ve en tu vida? Si es una virtud, ¿puedes identificarla en otras personas? Haz una lista de las personas que parecen haber logrado la paz consigo mismas y con el mundo que las rodea. Reúnete con ellos/as, "ausculta sus ideas"*

*y pídeles que compartan sus herramientas personales para lograrlo. Evita estar rodeado de individuos negativos que ofrezcan respuestas que impidan tu progreso.*)

2. In life, there are some things that you just cannot change, no matter how hard you try. Look at all the things that you can change mentally, emotionally, physically, financially, and socially. Learn when to cut your losses and detach from those who are harming your emotional well and internal peace. Create a daily and weekly plan to start eliminating those aspects that are damaging your life and substitute them for positive elements. Evaluate your progress on a weekly basis. (*En la vida, hay algunas cosas que simplemente no puedes cambiar, no importa cuánto lo intentes. Mira todas las cosas que puedes cambiar, ya sea mental, emocional, física, financiera y social. Aprende cuándo reducir tus pérdidas y separarte de las que están dañando tu bienestar emocional y tu paz interna. Crea un plan diario y semanal para comenzar a eliminar aquellos aspectos o elementos que están dañando tu vida y sustitúyelos por elementos positivos. Evalúa tu progreso semanalmente.*)

 ### Quote #2

"That poverty is better in peace, than in war, poor wealth."
   "*Que más vale pobreza en paz, que en guerra mísera riqueza.*"

Author: Spanish Saying, (I. Castro, personal communication, March 4, 2018).

 **Processing questions for the clients (Preguntas de proceso para los/as clientes)**

1. What is the author of this quote trying to say? What's the core meaning of it? (*¿Qué intenta decir el autor con esta cita? ¿Cuál es el significado principal de esto?*)

2. Peace, especially internal peace, can be subjective. However, internal peace is typically manifested by the way we conduct our daily business. Hence, are you able to differentiate when you mistreat others due to your own internal struggles? Cite examples and process them. (*La paz, especialmente la paz interna, puede ser subjetiva. Sin embargo, la paz interna generalmente se manifiesta por la forma en que llevamos a cabo nuestras actividades diarias. Por lo tanto, ¿puedes diferenciar cuando maltratas a otros/as debido a tus propias luchas internas? Citar ejemplos y procesarlos.*)

3. Homework: Turn off your phone, or at least silence it for 30 minutes to one hour. Select a time of the day that communication is not critical and will not affect your daily work responsibilities. Likewise, turn off the TV, radio, or any other electronic device that can distract you. Don't check your email on the computer or browse the Internet. Go outside, ideally where there is nature (i.e., park, beach, lake, river), and select a quiet place. Sit and feel the ground, grass, and plants. Close your eyes, breath in and out. Simply be in the moment. Experience the environment and just slow down. Once you have achieved a state of internal calmness, mentally start listing the things that are stealing your internal peace. Be specific and label them. Certain people, aspects of your work or business, current environment, phone, Internet, TV, residential area, etc. What can you do to modify your interactions with these on your list and how can you alter your

reactions toward these that are affecting your internal well-being? Remember that internal peace is not only a state of being but a choice of living. (*Tarea: apaga tu teléfono, o al menos silencialo de 30 minutos a una hora. Selecciona una hora del día en que la comunicación no sea crítica y no afecten tus responsabilidades laborales diarias. Del mismo modo, apaga la TV, la radio o cualquier otro dispositivo electrónico que pueda distraerte. No revises tu correo electrónico en la computadora o navegues por Internet. Sal fuera, idealmente donde haya naturaleza (es decir, parque, playa, lago, río) y selecciona un lugar tranquilo. Siéntate y siente el suelo, el césped y las plantas. Cierra los ojos, inhala y exhala. Simplemente siéntete en el momento. Experimenta el medio ambiente y solo disminuye tu velocidad. Una vez que hayas alcanzado un estado de calma interna, comienza mentalmente a enumerar las cosas que te están robando tu paz interna. Sé específico y etiquétalas. Ciertas personas, aspectos de tu trabajo o negocio, entorno actual, teléfono, Internet, televisión, área residencial, etc. ¿Qué puedes hacer para modificar tus interacciones con estos en tu lista y cómo puedes alterar tus reacciones hacia estos que están afectando tu bienestar interno? Recuerda que la paz interna no es solo un estado de ser sino una opción de vida.*)

### ·)) ⌂ Quote #3

"Who has peace in his conscience, has everything."
 "*Quien tiene paz en su conciencia, lo tiene todo.*"

Author: Giovanni Melchiorre Bosco, better known as Don Bosco. He was an Italian Roman Catholic priest, educator, and writer of the 19th century (Rodriguez, n.d.).

### ·)) ⌂ Processing questions for the clients (Preguntas de proceso para los/as clientes)

1. When during the day do you stop to evaluate your conscience? Do you ever evaluate your internal being? What is your standard or aspiration? How do you strive to be at peace with yourself? Explain. (*¿Cuándo durante el día te detienes para evaluar tu conciencia? ¿Alguna vez evalúas tu ser interno? ¿Cuál es tu estándar o aspiración? ¿Cómo te esfuerzas por estar en paz contigo mismo? Explica.*)

2. Describe the picture that follows. What are her feelings at this moment? Where is she? What is she trying to accomplish? What does it say about you? (*Describe la imagen de abajo. ¿Cuáles son tus sentimientos en este momento? ¿Dónde está ella? ¿Qué está tratando de lograr? ¿Qué dice esto sobre ti?*)

3. Take a piece of paper and attempt to draw something that represents peace according to you. Is this drawing a representation of an object, person, place, or event? Can this drawing be replicable frequently in your life? How can you accomplish this and what is preventing you from doing it? (*Toma un pedazo de papel e intenta dibujar algo que represente la paz según tu mismo/a. ¿Es este dibujo una representación de un objeto, persona, lugar o evento? ¿Puede este dibujo ser replicable con frecuencia en tu vida? ¿Cómo puedes lograr esto y qué te impide hacerlo?*)

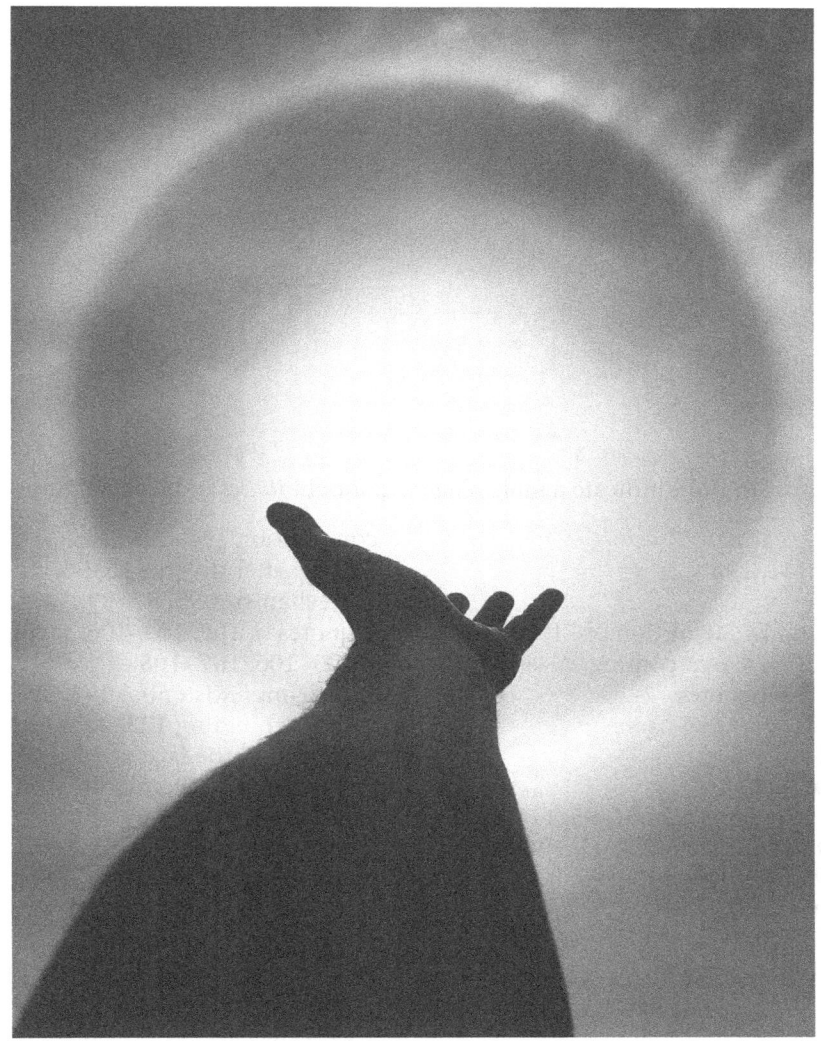

*Figure 22.1* Arms Outstretched to the Sky

## References

Rodriguez, C. (n.d.). *10 Don Bosco phrases to inspire young people for a better future.* ASHE. https:// ashepamicuba.com/en/frases-de-san-juan-bosco-a-los-jovenes/

Spinoza, B. (2021, February 11). www.goodreads.com/author/quotes/122092.Baruch_Spinoza

# Index

Note: Page locators in **bold** indicate a table. Page locators in *italics* indicate a figure.